CUTTING THE MONKEY-ROPE

CUTTING THE MONKEY-ROPE

John Galen McEllhenney

JUDSON PRESS, Valley Forge

HIEBERT LIBRARY
FRESNO PACIFIC UNIV.-M. B. SEMINARY
FRESNO, CA 93702

CUTTING THE MONKEY-ROPE
Copyright © 1973
Judson Press, Valley Forge, PA 19481

All rights reserved. No part of this publication may be reproduced, stored in a retrieval system, or transmitted in any form or by any means, electronic, mechanical, photocopying, recording, or otherwise, without the prior permission of the copyright owner, except for brief quotations included in a review of the book.

Except where otherwise indicated, the Bible quotations in this volume are in accordance with the Revised Standard Version of the Bible, copyright © 1946 and 1952, by the Division of Christian Education of the National Council of the Churches of Christ in the United States of America, and are used by permission

Other versions used are:

The New English Bible. Copyright © The Delegates of the Oxford University Press and The Syndics of the Cambridge University Press, 1961, 1971.

Today's English Version of the New Testament. Copyright © American Bible Society, 1966.

Library of Congress Cataloging in Publication Data
McEllhenney, John.
    Cutting the monkey-rope.
    Includes bibliographical references.
    1. Life.   2. Abortion.   3. Euthanasia.
I. Title.
BJ1533.H9M3   241   73-2550
ISBN 0-8170-0581-1

Printed in the U.S.A.

FOR NANCY

her love: a star

"We may take something like a star
To stay our minds on and be staid."
—Robert Frost

(from "Take Something Like a Star," by Robert Frost, *The Poetry of Robert Frost*, ed. Edward Connery Lathem [New York, Holt, Rinehart and Winston, 1969], p. 403. Copyright 1949, © 1969 by Holt, Rinehart and Winston, Inc. Reprinted by permission of Holt, Rinehart and Winston).

CONTENTS

1. The Monkey-Rope   11

2. Man Is Flesh   19

3. Fleshing-Out Man's Fleshliness   33

4. Four Attitudes Toward Dying   45

5. Subtilizing Our Minds   55

6. Distinctions and Acts of Extinction   67

7. Cutting the Monkey-Rope   77

8. Abortion   91

9. Euthanasia   105

Concluding Note: Monkey-Ropes   119

1. THE MONKEY-ROPE

Stretched taut between you, my reader, and me is a rope of plaited dreams. It cannot be seen. Neither can it be clutched. No skin at our waists is rubbed raw by its twisting. Yet this cord binds. It is a "monkey-rope" which links us together.

Such symbolic significance was given to the whaler's "monkey-rope" by Herman Melville in *Moby Dick*. After a whale has been harpooned and before the business of cutting in can begin, someone must insert a blubber hook in the giant carcass. To slip while doing so is to slide into shark-infested waters. Hence, a rope is attached to a canvas girdle worn by the man who climbs down to the whale's back. At its other end this hempen cord is tied to the leather belt of a sailor on deck. They are linked by the "monkey-rope."

After indicating the need for this protective line, Melville's Ishmael, calling the man slipping on the behemoth's spine by name, continues:

> . . . should poor Queequeg sink to rise no more, then both usage and honor demanded, that instead of cutting the cord, it should drag me down in his wake. So, then, an elongated Siamese ligature united us. Queequeg was my own inseparable twin brother; nor could I any way get rid of the dangerous liabilities which the hempen bond entailed.
>
> So strongly and metaphysically did I conceive of my situation then, that while earnestly watching his motions, I seemed distinctly to perceive that my own individuality was now merged in a joint stock company of two: that my free will had received a mortal wound; and that another's mistake or misfortune might plunge innocent me into unmerited disaster and death.

Therefore, I saw that here was a sort of interregnum in Providence; for its even-handed equity never could have sanctioned so gross an injustice. And yet still further pondering—while I jerked him now and then from between the whale and the ship, which would threaten to jam him—still further pondering—I say, I saw that this situation of mine was the precise situation of every mortal that breathes; only, in most cases, he, one way or other, has this Siamese connexion with a plurality of other mortals. If your banker breaks, you snap; if your apothecary by mistake sends you poison in your pills, you die.[1]

We humans are linked by a "Siamese ligature." Who I am shapes what I write. Everything I have thought and read and done influences my view of human life. And who you are determines how you interpret my intentions. You see my words but you hear your thoughts. Therefore, the freedom of each of us receives a "mortal wound." My desire to communicate is limited by the person you are. Your freedom to respond is limited by the way my materials are organized.

In a vital sense, however, this "monkey-rope" constricts me more than it does you. You can argue with me, but I cannot reply. Neither can I project at my writing table what you will bring to this book when you peruse it in one sitting, which is the procedure I suggest for the first reading. Circumstances make it impossible for me to know you. Were you an "unwanted" child? Advocates of legalized abortion say that one person in three was. Are you childless? The number of children available for adoption is decreasing. Has illness created a crisis of faith? Do you ponder the untimely deaths of productive persons and the unseemly lingering of the senile? Have you winked at some violent acts while shouting in righteous indignation at others? I will never know, but my inability to know what goes on in your mind should not keep me from sharing some of my formative experiences with you.

First of all, I like to people-watch. The ways in which personalities are brought out through choices of clothing intrigue me. This hobby's finest hour came one evening at the Philadelphia Museum of Art on the occasion of the gala opening of the Van Gogh exhibit. I stationed myself at the head of the grand staircase to watch those who were there to be seen. Establishment types promenaded in black ties and gowns from shops catering to the carriage trade. Antiestablishment types were wearing miniskirts, peasant dresses, jeans, and boots bought at boutiques. Caught between were those with shifting fashion allegiances.

Observing this parade, one of Thoreau's Walden-side musings came to mind: "Perhaps we should never procure a new suit, however ragged or dirty the old, until we have so conducted, so enterprised or sailed in some way, that we feel like new men in the old, and that to retain it would be like keeping new wine in old bottles."[2] How much old wine was sloshing about in new skins at the Van Gogh exhibit? Was I a new man in my new suit with the wider lapels? Doubtful. Most of us were giving visibility not to our inner selves, but to the dictates of the designers.

Styles change so that clothiers can increase their profits by selling new outfits before old ones wear out. Spring and fall fashion forecasts induce the feeling that one is about to appear obsolete. In the annual Easter Parade, there is much old life in new containers.

Something similar occurs in the idea market. New moralities are manufactured. They are promoted as harbingers of trends in human behavior. It is said of each intellectual fashion that it is an idea whose time has come. In some instances that assertion is true. More often the heralded moral fad is a familiar and rejected pattern imposed upon recently woven cloth. Old styles reappear, just as the recently popular long hair and shaggy beards have resurrected the romantic mood of the late eighteenth century. That movement was in reaction against the smooth-shaved intellectualism of the Enlightenment.

By now it should be obvious that I am suspicious of the fashionable in the field of ethics. When we are concerned with issues of life and death, the colorful new must not be allowed fashionably to replace ways of thinking which through usage have come to fit the form of human life.

Secondly, the guidelines proposed in this work are not divorced from my own emotion-charged experiences of life and death. What has happened to me is not unique. Neither are my encounters with life-arriving and life-departing capable of being universalized. They are mine. They have influenced my theorizing. And they must be reckoned with in reading this book.

The existence of one more human being is not a matter of indifference to me: My wife and I waited years for a child. At last, we were advised to adopt. We visited the agencies, studied the literature, and submitted applications. Months later we were invited to come and meet a little girl. Her big blue eyes chose us. Parental love was born.

Ten months after that baby girl gave birth to parental love, our marital love gave birth to a son. When I recount this experience, people say, "It happens often." It does, I know, but the *why* is shrouded in unknowing. And, where there is mystery, we ought not act as if we possess full knowledge. Reverence for life keeps us from making distinctions which permit acts of extinction. Specifically I cannot accept the argument that prenatal life is not human life. To distinguish thus is to permit abortions with an easy conscience. It is also to assume that we know more than we do about life in the womb. Where our knowledge is incomplete, a "monkey-rope" view of the world demands that we hedge our actions.

Not distant from the time of this writing my mother died. Her fatal illness was painful. Drugs were only partially successful in relieving the fierceness of her agony. Although many bodily systems were affected, her heart remained strong, thus prolonging the process of dying. Yet this suffering did not alter her essential personality. She would interrupt a bedside conversation in which she had evidenced no interest to ask if her grandson's bedroom furniture had been delivered. And flesh touching flesh remained an expression of love. Living through those months of my mother's dying, I learned that we must be circumspect about redefining death.

What taught me most, however, was our children's response to their grandmother's death. While her health was failing, they sensed something was wrong. She was too weak to get down on the floor with them to build "pigpens" with the blocks of my boyhood. They saw her once in the hospital. The wheelchair and the limpness of the hugs aroused concern, leading to questions about whether "Mommy Mac" was dying.

When the news of her death came, they were in bed. I waited until the following morning to tell them. They listened to my words and went back to playing. Then, when I least expected the question, they asked: "Why did Mommy Mac *have* to die?"

Centuries of human experience with dying were epitomized by the reactions of our daughter and son. Death broke into their daily activity, and they knew of nothing to do except to go back to what they were doing. Yet at the same time they vaguely recognized that dying belongs to the order of necessity: "Why did Mommy Mac *have* to die?" In the weeks that followed, random comments revealed that they had proceeded to the conclusion that their parents and even they themselves *have* to die. No adult grasps more about death than our seven-year-old and her brother. We may increase scientific information and improve medical procedures, but, when death comes, we can do no more than acknowledge its necessity and resume the daily round.

Just as my interest in clothing fashions makes me dubious of theological and ethical ones, so have my personal encounters with nascent and dying human life made me wary of cavalier attitudes toward life and death. Where there is uncertainty, it is best to fence behavior with those restraints that most adequately protect life. Many people today oppose capital punishment because there always remains the possibility that a legally condemned man is, in fact, innocent and that fresh evidence will come to light to effect his acquittal. If there is a shadow of a doubt, preference must be given to life.

Finally, at my end of our "monkey-rope," there is deference toward the ticking of clocks. Fresh from seminary, I was the associate pastor in a church where the Sunday services were broadcast live. Sermons had to conclude at 11:55 A.M., whether or not the preacher was finished. Watching my watch in the pulpit taught me to plan carefully. Not everything could be said that was thought during the hours of preparation. Some flights of fancy had to be shot down.

Likewise choices had to be made in writing this book. It might have been organized around population urgencies, beginning with the biblical fear of too few people and concluding with the contemporary fear of too many. Instead, I have concentrated upon individual human life. Abortion and euthanasia could have been treated in terms of the legislation that churchmen ought to favor. Instead, I have dealt with them as problems with which the consciences of Christians must wrestle. For the sake of saying some things as clearly as I can, other important considerations were left out.

In this book I shall employ the metaphor of the "monkey-rope" within the context of Melville's observation which has been cited: "I saw that this situation of mine was the precise situation of every mortal that breathes; only, in most cases, he, one way or other, has this Siamese connexion with a plurality of other mortals. If your banker breaks, you snap; if your apothecary by mistake sends you poison in your pills, you die."

Melville's vision of the interrelatedness of life remains fundamentally correct. Human existence is corporate. Man is man within a web of "monkey-ropes." What our twentieth century has added to the nineteenth-century novelist's insight is factual corroboration.

The Greenland Ice Sheet has been studied by Claire Patterson, a geochemist from the California Institute of Technology. By counting the annual layers of accumulation and by testing each for lead content, Patterson noted a fourfold increase in the amount of lead in the ice following the Industrial Revolution. After 1940, when lead began to be added to gasoline for automobiles, there was a frightening increase. Turning our attention to Antarctica, we learn that DDT sprayed on cotton fields in Arizona has been found in penguins, seals, and other animals.[3] When man seeks to increase his mobility or eliminate a competitor, he may ultimately kill a friend or himself. Deeds inspired by good motives often have evil hangers-on.

While not blinking the tragedies inherent in our "monkey-rope" world, neither dare we close our eyes to its glories. One of these has been reported by Jeanne Wellenkamp. She and her husband live in the middle of an apartment complex in Miami. One summer was unusually dry. Birds had trouble finding water. Noticing their plight, she put a saucer of water on the windowsill. Among the birds attracted was a cardinal. Soon he became a friend of the family, and sunflower seeds were added to the menu.

Observing developments, the reporter and her husband wondered if they were making a "welfare case" of this red bird. Some nights they withheld the seeds and discovered: "On the evenings we didn't put out refreshments, the little male cardinal would alight at our window and complain. He'd almost stamp his feet."

So linked was this bird to his human neighbors that the arrival of a phonograph record precipitated a crisis. It was a recording of Antonio Vivaldi's Concerto in C-major. There is a passage in this composition which imitates the song of the oriole. Jeanne Wellenkamp continues:

> One evening as we listened to this charming passage, we heard an angry peep at our window. There stood our favorite cardinal, not eating, not drinking, but glowering. He fluttered his crimson wings, tapped his rosy beak on the window. He appeared convinced that we had invited the oriole to live with us.[4]

If man is linked by "monkey-ropes" to the ice of Greenland, to the penguins of Antarctica, and to the birds on his windowsill, how much more is he tied to his fellowman! Testimony to this linkage is found in Cain's question: "Am I my brother's keeper?" (Genesis 4:9). No affirmative answer was thundered, but implicit in the whole transaction between Cain and God is a "monkey-rope" understanding of human life.

What was broken when Cain killed Abel was repaired in the life of Jesus Christ. Not only his words but also his actions bear witness to the responsibility of human life for human life. Even if Jesus had never talked about love of neighbor, that portion of the Great Commandment could be deduced from his example. Using the image of the vine and its branches, he established "monkey-rope" connections between himself and his followers. (John 15:5) Without doing violence to Jesus' intention in telling the parable of the good Samaritan, we can multiply these links of love to the point of visualizing a world in which each man is bound to every other man as securely as Queequeg was roped to his "Siamese twin" on the deck of the Pequod.

Just such a picture of life is assumed in this book. In brief, this is my thesis: Because human life is bound to human life in covenant relationship, nothing whatsoever *justifies* killing. On the other hand, there may be circumstances which render killing *exigent*, necessary, because God does not yet rule on earth as he reigns in heaven. Whenever such necessity is identified, however, it must not be justified as the "most loving" thing to do.

In the next chapter, the Hebrew view of man as flesh will be presented. Then, in chapter three, the manner in which medical research has enhanced our understanding of fleshly man will be examined. Learning how to be more precise about the moment of death does not make dying less terrifying. Chapter four deals with four attitudes toward life's terminus. In the next chapter we shall note how, through potlatch living, we may be courting destruction. The fact that violence produces nothing but violence is the theme of the sixth chapter, in which brain-created distinctions that incite acts of extinction are considered. Chapter seven deals specifically with the necessity on occasion for cutting the "monkey-rope." Those insights are applied to abortion in the next section and to dying in chapter nine. Finally, in the conclusion, I confess my debts in a "monkey-rope world."

2. MAN IS FLESH

At the bottom of a narrow flight of steps a door opened into a room I longed to enter: the Sistine Chapel. Head bent backward, I surveyed Michelangelo's ceiling, moving from the entrance toward the altar. A crick grabbed my neck. With that sharp pain came a mental process that led to spiritual insight.

Sitting along the wall with my eyes unfocused upon the floor, I began to realize what I had been looking at on the Sistine ceiling. Above the entrance, Noah is pictured as a sodden mass of flesh. The reason for his condition is apparent in the background. Taking advantage of God's rainbow promise, Noah had planted a vineyard. When the grapes ripened, he harvested them and tramped them into juice. One drink of the fermented beverage led to another until the man who had been lifted by God out of the mass of perverted human flesh fell into a drunken stupor.

The next panel reveals the destruction from which Noah had been rescued by the grace of God. Balancing a table loaded with cooking utensils upon her head, a woman tries to climb above the rising water. A man carries his wife piggyback; she looks back in terror at the onward rushing waves. Some swimmers attempt to clamber aboard the ark, but only those selected by God are safely settled in.

In a smaller scene, Michelangelo seems to suggest that Noah has found favor with God because he offered Him sacrifices, thus acknowledging that man lives in dependence upon the

Divine. Failure to be attentive to God has produced the situation portrayed in the center of the ceiling—Adam and Eve eat the forbidden fruit and are expelled, shamefaced, from the Garden of Eden.

The second half of my neck-twisting walk toward the papal altar began with God pulling Eve out of the side of Adam. That amusing panel is neighbor to one of the greatest scenes in the history of Christian art: the giving of life to Adam. Its focal point is a bit of empty space between the finger of God and that of Adam. Across that void moves the spark of life. Father God appears to hurtle toward the first man, simultaneously drawing Adam toward Him by infusing the material flesh of his being with the breath of life.

The artist's interpretation of this climactic moment is followed by paintings of three of the acts of creation which preceded it, namely, the gathering of the waters, the forming of sun and moon, and the separating of light from darkness.

It was obvious, of course, that I had shuffled from the ninth chapter of Genesis to the first in the course of moving from the entrance to the holy table. What slowly began to dawn upon me, as I relaxed, was what the sixteenth-century master was saying in the *way* he painted the scenes. Turning from the altar and reverting to the biblical sequence, the pilgrim sees the ceiling with spiritual eyes as he walks toward the door.

Where the Creator separates light from darkness, forms the sun and moon, and gathers the waters, his face is indistinct; it is not delineated clearly from the background. The features of God are not readily discernible. Michelangelo is saying that we get only an uncertain view of the Almighty in nature. The wonder of his works is there for us to behold, but we cannot look him in the eye. Hence we are unable to tell whether God's purpose in creating is spiteful or loving.

In the panel depicting man's creation, however, Adam's eyes focus upon a portrait-clear face of God. In forming him, the Maker's intention of having a creature capable of fellowship with Himself is revealed. This man is ideal humanity because in him flesh and spirit are harmoniously united. Totally attentive to God, the first man's flesh expresses the divine image pulsing within.

Unfortunately this flesh-spirit unity is soon broken. When

man ceases to pay attention to God, his flesh becomes a problem. No longer is it glorious in its nudity. Its nakedness is shameful. And the farther that the worshiper moves from the sacrificial table of the Sistine Chapel, the more do the figures on the ceiling sink into a fleshliness that is inexpressive of the image of God. Michelangelo's painting of Noah as a mass of besotted flesh marks the extremity of separation from God and the disharmony of flesh and spirit in man. What snores indifference to God more raucously than drunken stupor? Where other than in death itself is flesh less expressive of spirit?

Because Michelangelo was a genius in the genuine sense of that word, he may not have consciously worked out the scheme of his Sistine ceiling. Perhaps his inner eye glimpsed it as he meditated upon the Genesis accounts. In any case, what he left to posterity is a masterful portrayal of the continuum along which actual men can be located. All human beings find places somewhere between Michelangelo's Adam and his Noah. This fact was recognized in the Old Testament, and it is to this Hebrew view of human life that now we turn.

Old Testament man is flesh that is more or less expressive of what churns within. "Then the Lord God formed man of dust from the ground, and breathed into his nostrils the breath of life . . ." (Genesis 2:7). Man is enlivened dust. Man is flesh. Too often, however, the dustiness of man is skipped over to get more quickly to his spiritual qualities. Such haste is not encouraged by the Bible. There we find total involvement in the flesh.

This concentration upon fleshly life is easily misunderstood. Modern man thinks of flesh as being something he has too much of. Willingly would the person with an ever-expanding middle yield more than one pound to Shylock. Or modern man thinks of flesh in relation to the "Playmate" or the prude. Proponents of exposing more and more flesh to view are more successful than opponents of "skin flicks." Included in the opposition are persons who believe that "the world, the flesh, and the devil" are synonymous. Flesh to them is "worldly," and it is the devil who induces people to flaunt it. It is unfortunate that the element of truth contained in this argument blinds many to the Old Testament view of man.

Man *is* flesh. To be sure, God has breathed life into this flesh. But, in and of himself, man is nothing but flesh. "If [God] should take back his spirit to himself, and gather to himself his breath, all flesh would perish together, and man would return to dust." (Job 34:14-15) What *belongs* to man is the dust from which he was formed. But this flesh is not his burden; it is his glory. A "fleshless man" is unimaginable to the Hebrew for four reasons.

First of all, flesh makes the invisible "breath of life" visible. It shows us a person's thoughts and emotions. A scowl announces a storm within. This role of the flesh is similar to painting a picture. On the screen of his mind the artist's imagination projects an image. It is balanced. The colors harmonize. But it does not exist. Only when a canvas is set upon his easel and pigments mixed with oil are brushed over it, does what he saw come into view for others. The finished work of art is the flesh that reveals its creator's inspiration.

Looking at a painting, you and I assume that the eye's primary function is to take in what is external. That understanding of the eye is not foreign to the Old Testament, but a careful reading indicates that the eye is also a peephole through which others peer in at us. Eyes are like those slits in a fence about a construction site. They give one a chance to spy on the business at hand.

Eyes announce dissatisfaction. ". . . His eyes are never satisfied with riches . . ." (Ecclesiastes 4:8) and ". . . The eyes of a fool are on the ends of the earth" (Proverbs 17:24). There are "haughty eyes" (Proverbs 6:17) and humble eyes (Psalm 123:2), mocking eyes (Proverbs 30:17) and pitying eyes (Ezekiel 16:5). Eyes become "dim from grief" (Job 17:7), but they also lose their light when one's health is failing (Psalm 38:10). Once Jonathan was so hungry that his strength was ebbing. Coming upon honey, he put some to his mouth; immediately "his eyes became bright" (1 Samuel 14:27). The eye of flesh expresses what is happening behind that organ.

Flesh not only reveals what a man is thinking, the state of his health, and his contempt for or empathy with his brother, but it is also indicative of his attitude toward God. "O God, thou art my God, I seek thee, my soul thirsts for thee; my flesh faints for thee, as in a dry and weary land where no water is" (Psalm 63:1).

If a traveler in the desert does not come upon an oasis, his flesh dries up. So does the body of the pilgrim in the dry heat of God's absence. Flesh discloses that a spirit is suffering from a broken connection with God.

Second, flesh discloses to man the world in which he lives. Outer weather is carried inside. Each sense is a fleshly spy. Our ears hear the roar of minibikes and the songs of birds. Hands scratch in the dirt and caress soft faces. Eyes report on squalor and luxury. Noses sniff sulfur fumes and springtime. To our taste buds a carrot may be a delicacy, while caviar is simply too salty.

All senses link us to the world, but the ear takes precedence in the Old Testament. Through the other senses comes information, through the ear instruction. And it is more important for man to know how to act than merely to know. Hence the repeated stress on hearkening to God. "The Lord God . . . sharpened my hearing that I might listen like one who is taught. The Lord God opened my ears and I did not disobey or turn back in defiance" (Isaiah 50:4-5, NEB). The ears of man disclose a world in which the will of an invisible God is more to be heeded than the sight of an imperious majority.

In the third place, flesh enables man to control his world. It gives him mastery. Lacking it, he is powerless. There is a pen on my desk. My mind wills it to be grasped, but suppose my hands have been amputated. The intention has no fleshly instrument to carry out its will. No wonder then that the hand symbolizes power. Dante's Hugh Capet says: "I found that I held tight in my own hand the reins of state." With that grip on power came wealth. Hence, "tightfisted" long has been a description for the person who controls (and is controlled by) money. Medieval psychologists theorized that some demented persons would not unclench their fingers because they imagined themselves holding the whole world in their hands.

The hand is a biblical synonym for control. At the burning bush, God told Moses: "I have seen the affliction of my people who are in Egypt . . . and I have come down to deliver them out of the hand of the Egyptians . . . " (Exodus 3:7-8). Against God, Pharaoh is powerless. When man in his wholeness feels impotent, he implores: "Strengthen the weak hands . . ." (Isaiah 35:3).

That aspect of power which pertains to conquest and dominion is signified by the foot. Conquered kings were brought to Joshua following his victory made possible by the sun standing still at Gibeon. He ordered them to throw themselves at his feet. Then Joshua said to the chiefs of his men of war: "Come near, put your feet upon the necks of these kings" (Joshua 10:24). Man's responsibility for God's creation is stated thus by Psalm 8: "Thou hast given him dominion over the works of thy hands; thou hast put all things under his feet . . ." (8:6).

One of the strangest biblical euphemisms is the use of "foot" for the female genitals: "Thou hast . . . opened thy feet to every one that passed by, and multiplied thy whoredoms." (Ezekiel 16:25, KJV). Even here there is a suggestion of conquest.

Finally, it is through flesh that relationship is possible. Flesh is what men and animals have in common (Genesis 7:16 and 7:21). Preeminently flesh links man to woman: "Then the man said, 'This at last is bone of my bones and flesh of my flesh; she shall be called Woman, because she was taken out of Man.' Therefore a man leaves his father and his mother and cleaves to his wife, and they become one flesh" (Genesis 2:23-24). Flesh binds children to their parents. But there are fleshly ties with persons other than one's direct forebears or descendants. Laban is bound to his sister's son since Jacob is his own bone and flesh (Genesis 29:14). Abimelech sends this message to his mother's family: "Remember also that I am your bone and your flesh" (Judges 9:2). All the tribes of Israel said to David: "We are your bone and flesh" (2 Samuel 5:1). And David sent a message to the elders of Judah: "You are my kinsmen, you are my bone and my flesh . . ." (2 Samuel 19:12). Flesh is expressive of relationship, whether that most intimate one of husband and wife, or that which exists between animals and human beings.

Melville shows that he grasps this biblical understanding of the flesh at two points in *Moby Dick*. Captain Ahab has an artificial leg. Shattered in the chasing of a whale, he speaks to the ship's woodworker about fashioning another:

> Look ye, carpenter, I dare say thou callest thyself a right good workmanlike workman, eh? Well, then, will it speak thoroughly well for thy work, if, when I come to mount this leg thou makest, I shall nevertheless feel another leg in the same identical place with it; that is, carpenter, my old lost leg; the flesh and blood one, I mean.[1]

So completely is the limb of flesh part of one's concept of self that its amputation does not always eliminate the sense of its presence. Medicine calls this the feeling of the "phantom limb." At an earlier point in the tale, Stubb recounts a dream. In it Ahab kicked him with his artificial leg, but he did not take it as an insult, because "there's a mighty difference between a living thump and a dead thump. That's what makes a blow from the hand . . . fifty times more savage to bear than a blow from a cane."[2] Only flesh can give rage its fitting means of expression.

In company with Stubb, the Old Testament takes man's fleshliness with utmost seriousness. God created man by breathing into his nostrils a spirit that is expressed in and through congealed dust.

Attached to this fleshly man is a "monkey-rope" wound at its other end around the heart of God. There is a solemn agreement between God, whose footing is secure, and man. Regardless of the slipping and sliding of his partner, God will not cut the rope. When his "Siamese twin" gets himself in a jam, God does not set him adrift. He comes down in his wake.

This theme of God's love for irresponsible man is given classic expression in the sixteenth chapter of the Book of Ezekiel. God describes Jerusalem as the product of an Amorite-Hittite liaison. No one had tied her umbilical cord at birth. Instead she was abandoned to die. No eye but God's looked upon her with pity. He saw her and said to her, "Live" (16:6).

The fleshly sensuality of this chapter is heightened as God continues to speak. "You grew up and became tall and arrived at full maidenhood; your breasts were formed, and your hair had grown; yet you were naked and bare" (16:7). Jerusalem was ready for love. So God pledged himself to her and entered into covenant with her. He washed the blood of her shattered virginity from her thighs and anointed her skin with oil. Then God clothed her in silks and decked her with gold and silver. Reports of her beauty went out to all nations because of what God had done for Jerusalem.

But Jerusalem did not put her trust in God, who had bound

himself to her in covenant love. Rather, she trusted in her own fleshly loveliness and enticed passersby to sample what was pledged to God. She "played the harlot" (16:15). In this passage appears the euphemism that was noted previously: "Thou hast . . . opened thy feet to every one that passed by, and multiplied thy whoredoms" (16:25, KJV). Most prostitutes are paid for their favors, but not Jerusalem. She gave "gifts to all [her] lovers, bribing them to come to" her (16:33).

Such lewdness cannot go unpunished. God will gather all of Jerusalem's former lovers against her. "Because you have not remembered the days of your youth, but have enraged me with all these things; therefore, behold, I will requite your deeds upon your head, says the Lord God" (16:43). Jerusalem will suffer, but the "monkey-rope" will not be severed; she is not to be set adrift. "I will establish my covenant with you, and you shall know that I am the Lord, that you may remember and be confounded, and never open your mouth again because of your shame, when I forgive you all that you have done, says the Lord God" (16:62-63).

To speak more abstractly, there are two partners to this covenant: God, whose love is not elicited by man's worthiness, and man, whose worth exists only in the eyes of God. That man is not inherently worthy of God's love is obvious. We need only recall Noah. He is shown sprawled in immodest drunkenness in one colored woodcut. In the background, a goat rears up to munch grapes. This idea comes from a Hebrew legend which says that Noah learned the secrets of intoxication by watching a goat get drunk on wine. The man to whom God gave the rainbow sign played the goat.

What sort of a God would rope himself to a wastrel like Noah or to a whore like Jerusalem? What sort of a God would decline to cut such irresponsible and unlovable persons adrift? In the language of the Old Testament, he is a *redeemer* God.

In Israelite society, the *redeemer* was the person responsible for reclaiming the man who got himself in trouble. If a Hebrew found himself in debt to a foreigner, he might be forced to sell himself into slavery to that man. If that drastic step were taken, then it was incumbent upon his brother or uncle or cousin to buy him back, to "redeem" him (Leviticus 25:47-49). This reclaimer of bankrupt individuals was the redeemer.[3]

At some point, it was recognized by a person of insight that the Holy One of Israel behaved like a redeemer. When his people were enslaved by Pharaoh, He "redeemed" (Deuteronomy 24:18) them by commissioning Moses to lead them out of the land of Egypt. But God himself lent a hand. He sent a series of plagues, and he opened a path through the waters for the Israelites. All this concern was not drawn forth from God by deep-seated Hebrew worthiness. On the contrary: "Fear not, you worm Jacob, you men of Israel! I will help you, says the Lord; your redeemer is the Holy One of Israel" (Isaiah 41:14). Just as an uncle redeems his bankrupt nephew, so does God redeem his bankrupt people, that "worm Jacob."

In and through this act of releasing his people from Egyptian slavery, God made a covenant with them. He would continue to be their redeemer. In response to his gracious love, they would live their lives within certain boundaries. This relationship comes clear when we note that the root meaning of the word "covenant" is "fetter."[4] God binds himself to his people by the "monkey-rope" of love. This rope sets limits which we may think of as fences defining the behavior of the Israelites.

These fences are apparent when we look at those offenses punishable by death. They are idolatry, blasphemy, working on the sabbath, sorcery, the prostitution of a priest's daughter, intentional homicide, seizing a man to make a slave of him, striking or cursing parents, adultery, incest, sodomy, and bestiality. It may seem to us completely out of order to assess capital punishment in most, if not all, of these cases. Nevertheless, a logic operates here which reveals to us what the Israelites took seriously. Because a "monkey-rope" bound them to God, certain actions were prohibited. Capital punishment was not seen as a deterrent, but rather as a concrete witness to the holiness of life. Three categories of restrictions are discernible in this list.

First, priority is given to God and his worship. Idolatry (Exodus 22:20), blasphemy (Leviticus 24:16), and sorcery (Exodus 22:18) were punishable by death. The day of worship is fenced from profanation by capital punishment; "whoever does any work on the sabbath day shall be put to death" (Exodus 31:15). Since the priestly family line must be kept pure, burning is prescribed for a priest's daughter who becomes a prostitute (Leviticus 21:9).

Next, two offenses against the sanctity of life were punished by death. A murderer was to be executed (Exodus 21:12). No monetary ransom for his life could be accepted. The blood he had shed polluted God's land (Numbers 35:31-34). If a man should steal another man for the purpose of making a slave of him, that slaver was to be put to death (Exodus 21:16).

Finally, the human sources of life were protected. Children were to die for cursing or striking their parents (Exodus 21:15, 17). Adultery (Leviticus 20:10), incest (Leviticus 20:11, 12, 14, 17), sodomy (Leviticus 20:13), and bestiality (Leviticus 20:15-16) were capital crimes. If human beings are tied by a "monkey-rope" to God, then all is sacred that pertains to their coming into existence.

The preceding items are prohibitions, but this covenant relationship also included positive commands. God ordered his people to leap over certain of the fences that men delight in erecting. God "executes justice for the fatherless and the widow, and loves the sojourner, giving him food and clothing" (Deuteronomy 10:18). Because God loves the foreigner, he passes this injunction along the "monkey-rope": "You shall not oppress a stranger; you know the heart of a stranger, for you were strangers in the land of Egypt" (Exodus 23:9). Those familiar with what it is like to be away from home were to provide for the homeless. For strangers in their midst, they were to leave fallen grapes (Leviticus 19:10), and not to reap the edges of their fields (Leviticus 23:22). "When you beat your olive trees, you shall not go over the boughs again; it shall be for the sojourner, the fatherless, and the widow" (Deuteronomy 24:20). No questions were raised about the worthiness of these "welfare cases"; neither were there residence requirements.

God's love for the people of Israel was freely bestowed. It was not elicited by any inherent merit on their part. Therefore, God bound them to respond similarly to other strange people. Without strings they had received, without strings they were to give. The only string was the "monkey-rope" which bound man to God and to each of his neighbors.

Death cuts this "monkey-rope." Dead flesh cannot enter into relationship with living flesh. No control is exerted over the world by flesh that has lost its life-giving spirit. Nothing is less expressive of personality than a corpse. For the Old Testament, the end of fleshly life is death; nothing else.

From a perspective shaped by two thousand years of Christian history, it is not easy to grasp the Hebrew concept of death. We have been taught to think of the body returning to dust and the soul returning to God. But the Old Testament view of death is one of the breath of life departing from a fleshly man who will now descend, body and soul together, to Sheol, the place of silence and utter weakness. In the pit, the "monkey-rope" with the living is severed. So is that "monkey-rope" which links man to God. "Sheol cannot thank thee, death cannot praise thee; those who go down to the pit cannot hope for thy faithfulness" (Isaiah 38:18). Death separates man from God. "The dead do not praise the Lord, nor do any that go down into silence" (Psalm 115:17).

Let us now examine this ancient attitude toward death in some detail. It is equally possible for the Old Testament to speak of dead bodies and dead souls (Numbers 6:6 and Ezekiel 13:19, KJV). The breath of life departs at death (Genesis 35:18). What follows death is scarcely important. Job taunts God by saying that He will no longer be able to torment him because he will cease to be: "For now I shall lie in the earth; thou wilt seek me, but I shall not be" (Job 7:21). The psalmist utters a similar thought, with the difference that he hopes for a blessing before oblivion: "Look away from me, that I may know gladness, before I depart and be no more!" (Psalm 39:13). Jeremiah speaks of death as "perpetual sleep" (Jeremiah 51:39). What is most common appears to be the notion that flesh and soul go to Sheol in a weakened state. "Sheol beneath is stirred up to meet you when you come, it rouses the shades to greet you, all who were leaders of the earth; it raises from their thrones all who were kings of the nations. All of them will speak and say to you: 'You too have become as weak as we!'" (Isaiah 14:9-10).

If one can hope for nothing satisfying after dying, what constitutes a "good death"? For the natural end of fleshly life to be accepted without regrets, three conditions must be met. The normal span of life, first of all, must be attained. This length of life is defined variously. Genesis 6:3 refers to one hundred and twenty years; more familiar is the threescore years and ten of Psalm 90:10. To live that long is to die in peace.

"You shall go to your fathers in peace; you shall be buried in a good old age" (Genesis 15:15). Shakespeare's "ripeness" is determinative. "You shall come to your grave in ripe old age, as a shock of grain comes up to the threshing floor in its season" (Job 5:26).

Second, one must have children.

> At a peasant or Bedouin wedding in modern Palestine, a pomegranate is sometimes split open on the threshold of the house or at the opening of the tent: its grains symbolize the many children their friends wish them.
> In ancient Israel, to have many children was a coveted honour.[5]

These children carry on the family name. "Like arrows in the hand of a warrior are the sons of one's youth. Happy is the man who has his quiver full of them!" (Psalm 127:4-5). Sons protect an aged father, they ensure that his name will be remembered, and they give happiness. "Grandchildren are the crown of the aged, and the glory of sons is their fathers" (Proverbs 17:6).

Finally, decent burial is necessary if dying is to be faced with equanimity. According to de Vaux, honorable burial was thought necessary because "the soul continued to feel what was done to the body."[6] Tobit got into trouble with Sennacherib by burying the dead bodies of his fellow countrymen that were left lying outside the walls of Nineveh. He felt it to be an act of charity to bury them (Tobit 1:16-22).

Many times, of course, these conditions of a "good death" were not met for Old Testament men. Even today, only a few live for seventy years. According to United Nations' statisticians, there are only five countries in the world in which a male can expect to reach the biblical life-span: Sweden, Norway, Netherlands, Iceland, and Denmark; but there are forty-one nations in which a woman has that life expectancy, headed by Sweden with 76.5 years.[7] Others echo the lament of old: "I said, In the noontide of my days I must depart; I am consigned to the gates of Sheol for the rest of my years" (Isaiah 38:10).

The lack of a son was felt keenly. Women thought barrenness disgraceful. Rachel said to Jacob: "Here is my maid Bilhah; go in to her, that she may bear upon my knees, and even I may have children through her" (Genesis 30:3). Because he had no son, Absalom erected a pillar in the King's Valley to preserve the remembrance of his name (2 Samuel 18:18).

To lose that to which one has given life is to have part of one's self cut off. At the funeral of Alexander Tvardovsky, who had been forced out in 1971 as editor of a Russian literary magazine, the novelist Alexander Solzhenitsyn spoke: "There are many ways of killing a poet—the method chosen for Tvardovsky was to take away his offspring, his passion, his journal."[8] Without children, one cannot hope to live on.

Since "the soul continued to feel what was done to the body," not to be buried was to be cursed. The corpses of Jeroboam's followers were deliberately exposed to the teeth of dogs in the city; they were to be bird food in the open country (1 Kings 14:11).

All of the above possibilities meant that Old Testament man—and modern man also—could not be confident of a "good death." Therefore, he hungered for some assurance that death does not cut the "monkey-rope" binding him to God. Both in Amos 9:1-2 and Psalm 139:8, there are hints that God's hand reaches to Sheol. A more positive assertion appears in Daniel: "And many of those who sleep in the dust of the earth shall awake . . ." (12:2). At most, these references are "intimations of immortality," however. A clearer answer to the question of whether or not death cuts the "monkey-rope" linking man to God had to await a certain third day.

For the time being, the Hebrew definition of abundant life was fleshly. "Blessed is the man who fears the Lord, who greatly delights in his commandments! His descendants will be mighty in the land; the generation of the upright will be blessed. Wealth and riches are in his house . . ." (Psalm 112:1-3). Because there was no certainty that God could reach one in the grave, either to punish or to compensate for previous injustices, Old Testament men hoped for wealth and children and a long life.

3. FLESHING-OUT MAN'S FLESHLINESS

These are not cloudless days for doctors and undertakers. The latter are accused of cruising along the American way of death to the bank. They are charged with exploiting grief for gain. To judge from the yelps of pain, such comments rub exposed nerves.

Doctors live under a dark cloud of public suspicion. It is said that they make the United States a haven of hope for the rich man who is sick. But the poor man in the hospital is at the mercy of medical students gaining experience. The American Medical Association spends too much money protesting innocence to be convincing.

Muckraking criticism overlooks one vital fact. Physicians and morticians do preserve the biblical concern for man as flesh. They never lose sight of the body. A visit to the doctor's office begins not with a pencil and a psychological inventory but with a request to step on the scales.

Occasionally a funeral director friend of mine has refused to carry out the orders of the next of kin. They would ask him merely to take the body to the crematory and consign it to flames without ceremony. It was not in him to obey, so he would give me a call. He and I then placed the body in the hearse with dignity. Before cremation the two of us participated in a service in which it was acknowledged that the corpse, until recently, had bodied-forth a person. My friend feels that the remains of a fellow human being should not be treated with scorn.

My admiration for the positive is not meant to whitewash

the negative. Funeral bills are a scandal. Nine times as much is spent on burying the dead in the United States as on cancer research.[1] Even Mark 14:3-9 does not relax the pinch of that statistic. There Jesus rebukes those who grumbled that the woman who anointed him ought to have sold the ointment and given the proceeds to the poor. He distinguishes between a *gift* of love and a *work* of love. Gifts of love to the poor can be given at all times. But the work of love, in which one does what needs to be done to prepare the loved one for burial, is tied to a specific moment. The woman with the alabaster box read the signs of the times: her Master expects a criminal's burial; therefore she anoints him in anticipation and is commended.[2]

That commendation supports due respect for the flesh, but it does not justify huge bills based upon the slogan: "Nothing is too good for the loved one." There are selfish morticians. Nevertheless, just as selfishness in anyone is a distortion of the injunction to love one's self wisely, so self-seeking on the part of the undertakers is the dark side of something essentially human: respect for the flesh that once gave visibility to a personality.

What is true of morticians is even more true of physicians. They take man's fleshliness with utmost seriousness. Approach a doctor and he will pound the flesh, listen to its murmurings, and peer into its orifices. Roentgen's rays probe the flesh beneath the flesh. As a consequence, we moderns are able to flesh-out the Hebrew notion that man is dust enlivened by the breath of God.

Although they were well aware of the role of flesh, the biblical authors show little knowledge about conception and pregnancy. The speaker in the Wisdom of Solomon says: "I too am a mortal man like all the rest, descended from the first man, who was made of dust, and in my mother's womb I was wrought into flesh during a ten-months space, compacted in blood from the seed of her husband and the pleasure that is joined with sleep" (7:1-2, NEB). This "wise" man had trouble counting; others didn't: ". . . ask a pregnant woman whether she can keep the child in her womb any longer after the nine months are complete" (2 Esdras 4:40, NEB). What is most characteristic of Old Testament knowledge, however, is expressed in Ecclesiastes: "You do not know how a pregnant woman comes to have a body and a living spirit in her womb; nor do you know how God, the maker of all things, works" (11:5, NEB).

If they did not know the *how,* they could nevertheless feel quickening and see birth. Therefore, special significance was attached to these two events. It was at quickening, the first readily perceptible movement of the fetus in the womb, that a woman was sure that new life was taking shape within her. For centuries men continued to wonder when this life became ensouled. This speculation finally came to focus in the opinion of Aristotle. He asserted that the male embryo was animated by the spiritual soul forty days after conception; for the female fetus such animation occurred at eighty days.[3]

Birth was most important to the minds of the ancients, first of all, because it was so painful. ". . . every man's courage shall melt away, his stomach hollow with fear; anguish shall grip them, like a woman in labour" (Isaiah 13:7-8, NEB). How could any woman forget such agony? No wonder that high significance was attached to birth!

Because it was necessary to know the sex of a child before the name could be given, and since sex could first be observed at birth, there was a second reason for feeling that birth was a major dividing line in the life of a person. What happened at that moment previewed the destiny of the child. Coming forth from Rebekah's womb, Jacob grabbed the heel of Esau; that act determined his name and his nature as a supplanter (see Genesis 25:20-26 and 27:36). For all these reasons birth, rather than conception, was the moment when it could be said that another person stood in the midst of Israel.

Because the modern medical specialty of fetology pays attention to the flesh and its growth, we may have to revise the biblical emphasis on birth. There are points in the development of a human being more momentous than the divide between life in the womb and life in the light of day. Fetal development has been carefully charted.[4]

The first point on this chart is conception. During sexual intercourse, more than 200 million of the male's sperm are ejected into the female's vagina. They swim through the womb (uterus) into the Fallopian tube, the purpose of which is to convey ova (eggs) from the ovary to the uterus. If an ovum is in the tube, a sperm may fertilize it (conception).

For a sperm to fertilize an ovum, a change must take place in the sperm (capacitation). This alteration is thought to be produced by a substance in the uterus or Fallopian tube and to occur six to eight hours after intercourse. If sperm are not capacitated, or if a sperm does not fertilize an ovum within twenty-four hours after it has been discharged, both ovum and sperm lose their potential for creating life.

If conception does take place, then a zygote is created. This zygote is composed of twenty-three chromosomes from the mother and twenty-three from the father. Together they make up the forty-six chromosomes found in a normal cell of the human body. Of infinitely greater importance is the fact that these chromosomes carry the minute informational specks which determine what sort of person will develop. Unless this zygote later divides to produce a twin, no other person in the human race has had or will have just this combination of genetic materials. Hence, what is created at conception is unique (a once-for-all bit of life).

The second point on the fetal development chart covers the period from conception until the fourteenth day. After fertilization, the zygote begins to divide (mitosis) at the rate of approximately one division per day. Mitosis occurs in the Fallopian tube for seven days. During this time, it is impossible to determine whether or not a woman is pregnant.

About day eight, the zygote moves into the uterus. Contained on the chromosomes is an outline of the tasks to be performed. One pole of that sphere of dividing cells begins to dig its way into the lining of the uterus (implantation). This portion of the zygote becomes the trophoblast, which produces hormones that— cooperating with other aspects of the ovarian cycle—change the lining of the uterus to accommodate implantation. As a secondary effect, menstruation is normally stopped. Meanwhile, the other pole of the zygote is developing into what will become the embryo.

Here we must pause to examine two items of importance. During this early period in the uterus, the sphere of cells may divide to form identical parts (twinning). These may remain separate, eventuating in more than one embryo, or they may recombine. Therefore, although all that is essential for developing humanness is settled at fertilization, not until the second week is it determined whether there will be one, two, or more individuals.

Furthermore, the trophoblast burrowing its way into the uterine lining is clearly a parasite. It destroys some of the cells of the mother and takes nourishment from her blood. From it develops the placenta. Within the placenta one set of blood vessels goes to the woman, another to the child; they do not join. Oxygen, dissolved food, and waste matter slip from one to the other as they exist side by side.

Only after implantation is it possible to detect pregnancy. The hormones circulating in the mother's blood, produced by the growing zygote, offer the basis for a chemical test. Of course, a scraping (curettage) of the walls of the uterus would also, while terminating the pregnancy, produce evidence of implantation.

Our chart's third point begins after the second week when the zygote becomes the embryo (Greek for "swelling"). Between the third and fourth weeks, it is one-tenth of an inch long. Heart pumping occurs.

By the end of six weeks, the embryo's length is one-third of an inch. All internal organs are present in an elementary state. No bone, only cartilage, makes up the skeleton. If the mouth or nose is tickled with a hair at the seventh week, the embyro will flex its neck. Fingers have grown to the first joint.

The eighth week is an important divide within this third state of fetal development. The embryo changes its name to fetus (Latin for "young one"). Electrical activity of the fetus's brain is readable. Fingers and toes are fully recognizable. Between the ninth and tenth weeks, swallowing, squinting, and other reflexes appear. Soon X-rays will show clear details of the fetal skeleton. The two-and-one-half-inch-long fetus now sucks its thumb. Electrocardiographic techniques pick up the fetal heart via the mother at week twelve.

Some time between the twelfth and the sixteenth week, quickening occurs. Much significance was attached to quickening in former days because it was the first moment when the woman could feel life within her. It remains important to the mother, but is insignificant insofar as fetal development is concerned.

By the twentieth week, the fetal heart can be heard by the simple stethoscope. A one-pound recognizably human fetus exists in the womb.

We move on to the fourth point in our developmental chart

with the twentieth week. Between then and week twenty-eight, a fetus born has a 10 percent chance of survival. These odds improve as time passes.

During the average of 266 days between fertilization and birth, that initial single-celled zygote develops into a complex 200-million-celled being. The blueprint for this development was there when the maternal and paternal chromosomes came together.

From the perspective of fetal development, birth is not especially important. Previously the fetus took oxygen from the mother; now he or she takes it from the air. Previously the fetus cried without tears flowing; now they begin to ooze. Of more developmental significance is the time about age one when the infant begins to use words.

Paul Ramsey notes:

> Before that, an infant is likely only potentially human by the standard of self-awareness or incipient rationality . . . (A)bout this time *full* cortical brain activity is achieved, as evidenced by the appearance of *rhythmical* markings on an electroencephalogram. Otherwise, brain and heart activity as signs of life have been evident long before birth.[5]

It is impossible to underestimate the content added by fetology to the biblical understanding of man as flesh. Now we *do* "know how a pregnant woman comes to have a body . . . in her womb" (Ecclesiastes 11:5, NEB). We have charted fetal development from the moment ovum and sperm combine. In chapter eight, this chart will be examined again in relation to the question of abortion. For now it stands as testimony to the wonder that is man and to the necessity of including the findings of medical science in one's Christian view of human life.

What medical science does not tell us is *why* "a pregnant woman comes to have . . . a living spirit in her womb" (Ecclesiastes 11:5, NEB). Before that question the scientist stands mute.

Biblical authors knew that man is flesh, but they often attached what are to us farfetched roles to his organs of flesh. Consider the human kidney. Its physiological function was unknown, but it was felt to be vital. Due to their color and density, animal kidneys were considered, along with the blood, to be at the center of life. Therefore, they belonged in a special manner to the deity and were offered to him in sacrifices.[6]

The King James Version translates the Hebrew word for kidney with *reins,* which derives from the Latin term for the organ. There are times when this word is used to describe the physiological kidney. "His archers compass me round about, he cleaveth my reins asunder, and doth not spare; he poureth out my gall upon the ground" (Job 16:13, KJV). In other places, the reins are the seat of the emotions. "Thus my heart was grieved, and I was pricked in my reins" (Psalm 73:21, KJV). The kidneys rejoice (Proverbs 23:16, KJV). It is also the role of the reins to instruct one in right behavior. "I will bless the Lord, who hath given me counsel: my reins also instruct me in the night seasons" (Psalm 16:7, KJV). God is in the mouth of the wicked but not in his reins (Jeremiah 12:2, KJV). There is no etymological connection between the biblical *reins* and the identical word which means a strap for controlling an animal. Nevertheless, both constrain.

This constraint was at the heart of Michel de Montaigne's musings on his kidney stones. He writes that his imagination says that it is

> for my good to have the stone; that the structure of my age must naturally suffer from some leakage. This is the time when they begin to loosen and decay. Such is the common lot. Would I have a new miracle performed in my favour? In this way I am paying the dues of old age, and I cannot expect to get off more cheaply.[7]

The pain of kidney stones led Montaigne not to seek obliviousness through drugs, but to thoughtfulness.

> If you tell me that the disease is dangerous and mortal, what diseases are not? . . . you do not die because you are sick, you die because you are alive. Death can easily kill you without the help of the disease. And sickness has postponed death for some people who have lived longer because they thought they were dying.[8]

Montaigne felt that the stone in his *reins* instructed him. Although he was not clear about the relationship, he knew that his kidneys were tied to his organ of sexual pleasure. Because that was the area of life in which his transgressions were greatest, his punishment seemed to be appropriate. Yet it was tempered. The agony came when he was too old to delight in sex.

When this French sage turned to describing *how* kidney stones develop, he knew little more than the ancients. His assumption was that age reduces the stomach's heat. Hence, more crude matter is passed on to the kidneys. They in turn lose their heat, so that what once would have been dissolved now hardens. And the only remedy available, Turk's herb, is ineffective.

Modern medical science reduces all these former thoughts about the kidney to one simple definition: "Either one of two glandular bodies in the lumbar region which secrete the urine."[9] Stones are "crystalline concretions of calcium oxalate, calcium phosphate, uric acid, or cystine."[10] When the sufferer fails to pass the stones, surgery provides relief.

For centuries, men endured the excruciating pain which *The Merck Manual* describes as radiating "across the abdomen and into the groin, genitalia and inner aspect of the thigh. The agony and writhing of the patient are extreme."[11] Montaigne writes about the "sharp rough-edged stone that cruelly pricks and tears the neck of [the] penis"[12] with equal exactness. But the French sage knew of no cure. Now there are specific treatments because physicians continued to pay attention to the flesh. They did not stop experimenting after reading Montaigne's *Essays*. From their philosophizing, physicians did not draw the conclusion that pain makes one think; thus, since thinking makes one wise, let pain prevail. No, they pursued ways of making life in the flesh more comfortable. And we are indebted to their perseverance.

In spite of that debt, medical science has not improved upon Montaigne's *attitude* toward illness. No technique has been devised for infusing the modern sufferer with his insights.

> Here is the proof of what I say. Since I last wrote, this new development has taken place, that the slightest movement draws the pure blood from my kidneys. What of it? I do not for all that give up moving about as before, and I gallop after my hounds with a youthful ardour that is unusual in me.[13]

Medicine knows how to treat a stone in the flesh. That was unknown to the Old Testament writers and Montaigne. But medicine does not know *why* one spirit bodied-forth by flesh reacts so differently to pain from another spirit.

What the Hebrews believed about a "good death" was noted in the previous chapter, but the means available for determining that death had occurred were primitive. One could wait until it was evident that this flesh no longer made the invisible "breath of life" visible—that it no longer carried sensations inward from the world—that it was now powerless—that relationships with other persons which it had once effected were broken. A body that no longer did these things was dead.

Rather than waiting to make certain that these four functions of the flesh had ceased, there were two rough-and-ready indicators related to the Old Testament concept of life. "And the Lord God formed man of the dust of the ground, and breathed into his nostrils the breath of life; and man became a living soul" (Genesis 2:7, KJV). Therefore, when there was no breath in the nostrils (Genesis 7:22), the person was dead. Whether or not there was breathing could be observed by watching the chest. Holding a mirror at the mouth would reveal even slight exhaling. The other test was tied to Leviticus 17:14—". . . for the life of all flesh is the blood thereof . . ." (KJV). If the blood was gushing out, the person was dying. When no movement of blood could be detected, or when the body became cold (2 Kings 4:34), death had come.

These indicators remained the principal ones down to the present century. The stethoscope enabled the physician to hear more acutely, but he still listened for the beat of the heart as did his counterpart of old. What has been added in the twentieth century is technology for measuring the electrical activity of the brain. Such measurements are recorded on an electroencephalogram. When the line on that piece of paper is flat rather than jagged, the brain is dead. Following brain death, the heart will continue to beat naturally for some time. However, when the brain dies, the lungs soon stop functioning. Oxygen is not supplied to the blood. Without oxygen the heart ceases to beat. A human being has died.

In addition to employing the EEG (electroencephalograph) for detecting brain death, modern medicine has developed ways and means for maintaining respiratory activity after the brain is dead. A respirator keeps the blood stream oxygenated. As a result, the heart continues to pump. The two traditional indicators of life, breathing and heartbeat, remain even though the electroencephalogram shows that the brain no longer lives.

Whether or not it is good to employ the respirator when there is no electrical activity in the brain will be discussed in chapter nine. For now, it is enough to draw attention to the fact that all of these highly sophisticated means for maintaining life (or prolonging dying) tend to isolate the dying person from other human beings.

Rules of intensive care units permit family members to visit five minutes each hour. Machines curtain off the patient. He is little more than the central link in a vast network of gadgets. "Where nature has failed, machines are succeeding. There are devices to breathe for patients who cannot breathe, to feed those who cannot swallow, to cleanse the blood of those whose kidneys have failed, to ring for help for those who cannot cry out."[14]

Motivated by the laudable intention of doing everything possible to save life, physicians are increasing the terrors of dying. No machine has a hand of flesh to clasp a weakening hand.

Morticians, desiring to spare feelings, hang a curtain of professionalism and cosmetics between dead flesh and living flesh. They care for the corpse. Their skills are employed to make that which has ceased to body-forth personality look the way it did when spirit was throbbing within. Lifeless flesh is not granted a dignity of its own.

Physicians take dying out of the home. Morticians assume responsibility for caring for the corpse. Their intentions are to provide better care for the dying and to decrease the anguish of the bereaved. With these demons driven out, however, there is emptiness (Matthew 12:43-45). Into the void rushes the fear of death.

At one time, I thought it was good that children would no longer go through what I did as a ten-year-old when my Uncle Perry died. We drove from our home to that of his widow, daughter, and son-in-law. After we arrived, the undertaker brought the coffin back into the living room. There it was opened and remained open. People came and went. Food was carried into the house. Tears flowed, since there was no way of ignoring what had happened. Just inside the front door lay the flesh which once had embodied a spirit that had been part of my life as long as I could remember.

I slept in the same house with a corpse. The next morning, Uncle Perry's funeral service was conducted where he lived.

Together we left that place to drive across town and up the hill to the cemetery.

Darkness covered my family's return journey that evening. I had time to think. There was no way for me to blink the fact that my favorite great-uncle had died. Was that confrontation beneficial? For many years I was not certain. In seminary I came to the conclusion that such funeral practices are pagan. That feeling remains with regard to using cosmetics and some other customs. But now I believe that I am less fearful of dying because Uncle Perry's death was so concretely experienced.

The funeral rites of ancient Israel will help us to grasp why death loses some of its sting when we look it in the eye.[15] When a Hebrew died, his eyes were closed, and the nearest relative embraced the flesh which only minutes before had made relationship possible. Usually burial took place that day. Until that moment the corpse remained in the house. These practices highlighted the fact of separation.

For the loved ones, the day of death and those that followed constituted a time of transition. Death had shattered their routine. Normal social activities were impossible. Even the daily round of preparing meals came to a stop. Neighbors and friends brought bread and the cup of consolation for those not fasting.

At the news of death, relatives tore their garments, put on sackcloth, and fasted. Because the wearing of sackcloth and fasting were part of the rite of penitence, these actions were concrete ways of dealing with guilt. Our forefathers recognized that at a time of loss there is always a gnawing doubt: Did I do all that I could have done? Mourners wore sackcloth to scratch the skin, and they disciplined their hunger. By so doing they neutralized the acids of guilt which, if left unalkalized, would bite the heart.

According to Roland de Vaux,

> The chief funeral ceremony was the lamentation for the dead. In its simplest form it was a sharp, repeated cry, compared . . . to the call of the jackal or the ostrich. . . .
> These exclamations of sorrow could be developed into a lament . . . composed in a special rhythm.[16]

Such cries enabled the mourners to pour out the emotion that bubbled inside.

With burial, dust returned to dust (Genesis 2:7; 3:19). And those who were already in Sheol stirred themselves to greet the newcomer (Isaiah 14:9-10) and to incorporate him into the realm of the dead. He was completely separated from the living.

But the rite of transition for those who were yet alive was not ended. Some action must mark the return to routine. Usually this was a celebrative meal eaten with one's relatives and friends.

There was a parallel to each of these Hebrew practices in what I went through when Uncle Perry died. The body in the house left no doubt in my mind that he was dead. Flowing tears gave expression to grief and, to some extent, to guilt. Burial made the return of dust to dust visible. The family meal back at the house, served by friends and neighbors, closed the gap which had appeared in the family circle. And, strange yet true to say, my brooding on those events left me not afraid of death but aware of my own mortality.

Continuing medical research has fleshed-out the biblical view of man as flesh. We now know more about pregnancy, illness, and dying than was imaginable to the ancients. Yet that knowledge has not solved the question of the meaning of birth, sickness, and mortality. In fact, the monkey-ropes which bind persons to each other at these critical moments may be less clearly discerned today. We isolate the sick. We camouflage death. Children are not allowed to see it. A curtain is drawn around it. Because what is not seen provokes fear and what is hidden provokes curiosity, death is a specter that both pushes away and draws one on. To man's responses to the ambiguity of death we now turn.

4. FOUR ATTITUDES TOWARD DYING

"A womb with a view"—that was the crow's nest of Dylan Thomas. Tailored by Cyril Connolly, this descriptive phrase fit the Welsh bard exactly.[1] Thomas needed to see the forms of the world in order to give shapes to his dreams. But, when it came to living in that world, he craved caressing care.

She who carried Dylan in her womb coddled him. His mother's way of rearing him produced an adult who was at a loss in dealing with clean shirts, publishers, and what bookkeepers keep records of: pounds and pence. His father opened to him an outlook on the world. He read from Shakespeare and stocked one room of their Swansea home with books. That hometown in Wales was uniquely situated to offer a view to a poet. As a seaport, Swansea stood between land and water, but it could not always provide all the sights Thomas sought. London did. So later did New York. Cities gave him perspective. Their sounds gushed into a mind that twisted them and then stretched them into rhythms that sounded his depths. But the noises of unfamiliar places sent Dylan, sooner or later, scurrying for a womb.

The problem is that, for the man born, only the tomb proffers that complete freedom from care that was enjoyed in the womb. Hence Dylan Thomas was pulled toward death. To be in the tomb was to be at peace. At peace, yes, but also in the dark. The child in the womb sees nothing. So the man who values perspective fears the tomb. It cuts off the view. This dread of death and its previously mentioned attraction produced alternating currents in Thomas's brain. And that electricity yielded one of his finest poems, "Do Not Go Gentle into That Good Night."[2] Written in May, 1951, the lines are addressed to the poet's father, who, because he was dying, never heard them. Dylan urged his sire to resist death because his words had sparked no fire, because his actions had been lifeless, and because his eyes had been dim. Watching D. J. Thomas go blind, Dylan cried to him to be angry with the approaching darkness. These are a son's thoughts while living through his father's dying. They are also the words of a poet who wondered if he too were a failure.

David John Thomas, father of Dylan, had wished to be a poet but lacked the gifts. To forget his dream, he drank. Drinking too heavily, he failed in his career as a teacher. Talking was all that was left; then cancer chewed at his tongue. Because he had lost out, he wished his son to succeed.

That son was troubled in May, 1951. Was he slipping toward death without having succeeded as a poet? His writings earned scant support for his family. His eyes were dulled by drink. No light shines in the grave, so he admonished himself—as well as his father—to rant against the Grim Reaper.

Thus speaking, Dylan Thomas gave contemporary expression to the Old Testament attitude toward death. To die was to descend to the domain of shadows. There flesh is weak. There it lacks all potential for making visible the breath of life. Death comes as the Great Dispossessor. It takes all that is essential. Eyes stop blazing, hands cease doing, words don't resound, and amassed wealth is useless. Jesus made that point in Luke 12:16-21, where he pictured death as the Great Dispossessor. A man built great warehouses for his possessions and said: "Soul, thou hast much goods laid up for many years; take thine ease, eat, drink, and be merry" (Luke 12:19, KJV). That night death took all. Fearing this deprivation, Dylan Thomas raged against death.

Death is the Great Dispossessor, but life has many small ones, reminders of the Great One. There is the old Hebrew list: "Four are compared with a dead man: the lame, the blind, the leper and the childless."[3] Whenever flesh loses one of its functions, the man of flesh sees a preview of death. Arthritic hands herald dead ones. Paralyzed lips point to a time when kissing stops. Hardened eardrums vibrate a warning that there is a soundless place. Old Testament man went reluctantly to Sheol; modern man rages against death.

This fear that there is no worthwhile life after the coming of the Great Dispossessor is not the only ancient attitude toward dying which is still current today. There are modern Stoics who embody what Melville calls "enormous practical resolution in facing death."[4] Montaigne looked that small dispossessor—a kidney stone—in the eye and commented with detachment: "If you do not embrace death, at least you shake hands with it once a month; and this gives you greater reason to expect that one day it will catch you without warning."[5] He saw kindness in the fact that illness drained him of life. "The final death will be so much the less complete and painful; it will kill no more than a half or a quarter of a man."[6]

Cato the Younger was the classic Stoic. He and his allies were defeated by Caesar in 46 B.C. With a small division Cato fled to Utica. Caesar followed. Deciding that defense of the city was impractical, Cato gave money to those who planned flight and suggested that his son yield to Caesar. For himself, he chose to spend the evening in conversation. Later in his room, Cato read Plato's description of Socrates' quaffing of the hemlock. His friends suspected that he planned suicide, so they took his sword. But, when they relaxed their watch, Cato ordered his servant to bring it back. With "enormous practical resolution," he shoved it into his abdomen. Alerted, the companions summoned a physician to dress the wound. Cato imitated sleep. His watchers left. Then he removed the bandages, tore out the sutures, pulled at his intestines, and died. Life no longer appealed to the great Stoic. Deliberately he determined to die.

With similar determination, John Berryman jumped off a bridge in Minneapolis onto the frozen Mississippi. Before he took that plunge, he turned and waved. It was January, 1972, and Berryman had just finished reading in proof the poems to appear in *Delusions, Etc.* In that book he submitted his resignation. What he wanted to say was said. He desired nothing, hoped for nothing. Because there was no one to sing for and nothing to sing about, Berryman displayed "enormous practical resolution in facing death."

Death is a womb-like darkness sought by some as preferable to life. They go into it with a wave, a flourish. And they do so unsupported by any belief in a place where singing shall be possible once more. Less than a whole person while drawing breath, they feel that little is left for death to claim.

Melville refers to a third group who assume an attitude of "speculative indifference as to death." These are they who believe in the immortality of the soul. Flesh is merely the housing of the soul. More, it is the spirit's jail. Therefore death is the warden who signs a writ of release. This notion of the soul's immortality can be traced back through the writings of eighteenth-century philosophers and the philosophizing of Christian thinkers to the teachers of ancient Greece. Associated with this theory that there is a part of man which automatically survives the Great Dispossessor is the belief that the soul will be rewarded or punished.

A three-thousand-year-old papyrus illustration in the Pierpont Morgan Library depicts Egyptian speculation on the question of judgment. One of the gods holds the balance; another records the results. The essence of the deceased is in one of the scales; in the other is a feather, symbolic of the lightness of purity. The dead man defends himself saying: "I have caused no one to weep, I have made no one suffer. . . . I have not taken the milk out of the mouths of children, nor have I driven cattle from their pasture. . . . I am pure, I am pure, I am pure."[7] Seldom is self-assurance expressed so bluntly, but presumption of innocence before the Final Tribunal underlies the "speculative indifference" of many "as to death." They anticipate a happy hunting or contemplating or playing ground on the other side.

Listen to the Masonic burial ritual in the twentieth century and you will hear the ideas of ancient Greece and Egypt dressed in the garments of eighteenth-century deism. Man's soul is immortal by nature. Death sets it free to go before an objective judge. Souls that are pure will be rewarded. Ones heavy with suffering provoked, tears elicited, and milk withdrawn will be tormented. But, like the Egyptians of old, few expect to outweigh a feather. If not to be overheard, at least in the gut of presumption they cry, "I am pure, I am . . ., I. . . ."

Raging against the coming of darkness, going with "enormous practical resolution" into the grave, and speculating about the soul's immortality: these modern approaches to dying are likewise antique. Some things never change under the sun. Yet, how they differ from the attitude of Jesus! He did not rage against death. Neither did he encounter it "with enormous practical resolution." And not as an immortal soul did Jesus appear to Mary in the garden.

Let us begin with that appearance. Mary first thought that the man behind her was the gardener (John 20:14-16). Then he spoke her name, and she heard her Master. Mary saw the Risen Lord. We must credit the account, since it is unlikely that the early church would invent a story in which a woman was the sole eyewitness. "Women were not qualified to give testimony."[8] Thus, if her report was respected in her day, we must respect it. And what she saw was a resurrected person, not an immortal soul.

In painting this scene, artists traditionally show the nail prints and the spear prick on the glorified body of Christ. By so doing, they make visible the insight of Paul: "When the body is buried it is mortal; when raised, it will be immortal. When buried, it is ugly and weak; when raised, it will be beautiful and strong. When buried, it is a physical body; when raised, it will be a spiritual body" (1 Corinthians 15:42b-44a, TEV). The New Testament views the other side of death in terms of a changed body. No support is given to the theory that the soul shakes off its shell.

Paul struggled to find language to convey this reality. It remains difficult to picture the resurrection, but Charles Barker has a painting which helps. To be helped, however, one must understand the symbolism of the automobile in his work. The car, like man, is a creature which threatens to dominate its creator. Cars are made by man and for man, but they appear on the brink of enslaving him. He is being strangled by the coils of their roads, suffocated by their exhaust, and beggared by their cost. Man was created by God and for God, but he seeks to bend God to his purposes. Seeing that parallelism, we come to understand that the automobile and its component parts stand for man in Barker's paintings.

In *Resurrection,* he uses tires. They are red and yellow. They soar toward the top of the canvas where they become transparent to the blue of the sky. Yet they are obviously tires: transformed tires, glorified ones to be sure, but tires. No longer are they black. Now their colors sing. So it is with the resurrection of man.

Now we are ugly, old bodies; then we shall be beautiful ones, transparent to the blue of God's truth. The Bible does not endorse "speculative indifference as to death." Neither is the judgment described by Jesus in Matthew 25:31-46 similar to that of ancient Egypt or eighteenth-century deism. Beside a pyramid the soul cried, "I am pure." Before the Good Shepherd the saved inquire with surprise, "When saw we thee sick, or in prison, and came unto thee?"

Second, Christ did not exhibit "enormous practical resolution in facing death" in the Garden of Gethsemane. Montaigne's bloody urine made him philosophical about dying. Looking at the cup held out to him to drink to the dregs, Jesus' sweat became tinged with blood. Since the time of Aristotle, such bloody perspiration has been noted occasionally under "conditions of extreme mental strain."[9] The agony of Jesus as he faced death was intense. Why? He understood that the kingdom of God comes through suffering. God is revealed in and through suffering. That is the point made in Isaiah 53. Jesus applied it to himself. But to understudy the role of suffering is quite different from playing the role. The human Jesus was tempted to avoid suffering. Like us he backed off.

Anger often manifests internal conflict. With that in mind, we can look at Mark 8:31-33. There Jesus talks about the suffering which he anticipates as a *must*. It is necessary for him to suffer, be rejected and killed. To this announcement of the necessity of suffering Peter objects. Now if Jesus were completely settled in his own mind concerning the *must* of his passion, we would expect him to reason with Peter as he later reasoned with the disciples on the Emmaus road. But Jesus barked at Peter. He called him "Satan." By so doing he revealed that he was not approaching dying with "enormous practical resolution." He was torn internally.[10]

In the end, however, Jesus did not rage against the coming darkness. His words had clout. He spoke and men saw. His eyes flashed and men heard. His deeds evoked dancing. Therefore, he could accept God's will. Hanging between heaven and earth, Jesus cried with a loud voice and said, "Father, into thy hands I commend my spirit" (Luke 23:46, KJV).

In and through his dying, Jesus made of suffering a gift. Job and his coreligionists experienced suffering as a problem. They believed that God rewarded the good with health and the bad with illness. Therefore, when they looked at specific instances in life, there was a problem to solve. Evil men enjoyed fullness of health. Good men were tormented in the flesh. Righteous Job sat on the ash heap and scraped his boils. Why do the unrighteous prosper and the upright go bankrupt? Suffering was problematic.

Suffering was also a scandal to some ancients. Philosophically minded Greeks and Romans could not fit suffering into an orderly world view. They reasoned thus: A good God, who was also powerful, would not allow suffering. Since suffering prevails, either God is good and weak, or strong but cruel. This attitude comes through in the oldest known depiction of the crucifixion. It is a graffito found on the wall of a villa on Rome's Palatine Hill. A stick man lifts his arms in adoration of the figure on the cross. The scribbled inscription reads: "Alexamenos worships God." What is shocking is the representation of the crucified one; he has the body of a human being but the head of an ass.[11]

We may conjecture that Alexamenos, a Christian, worked in a wealthy household. His fellow servants, holding to Greek notions about suffering and God, thought him a fool. How can God be disclosed in and through unmerited agony and death? "Ha!" they laughed; "Our cohort adores a donkey-like God." They were both right and wrong. Right—in seeing that the suffering one is focal for the Christian. Wrong—in that their theories made it impossible for them to discover love and power in pain.

Christians interpreted this suffering as a gift: the gift of forgiveness. They remembered the word from the cross, the syllables pushed out by lungs collapsing: "Father, forgive them; for they know not what they do" (Luke 23:34, KJV). They saw suffering; they felt forgiveness. It was not clear how the joining of these two occurred, but the consequence was certain: true believers became more truly human.

Rightly viewed, suffering humanizes. By the summer of 1940, the carvings of the artist Henry Moore had become abstract. He sculptured geometric patterns. Then came the London blitz. One mid-September evening, Moore and his wife had dinner with friends in Chelsea. Because gasoline was rationed, they took the underground.

When they reached the Hampstead Station on the return trip,

the doors of the tube train slid open and they stepped onto the platform with difficulty. Sleeping bodies littered it. What the Moores did not know until that moment was that Hampstead was one of the deepest underground stations in the metropolitan area. People came from great distances to sleep there in safety. Henry Moore's eyes were opened. Out came his sketch pad. Standing in a shadowed corner, he sketched reclining men and women. He returned night after night, leaving with reluctance when the all clear sounded. As a result, the human form returned to Moore's art. Suffering humanized him.

Christ's suffering does that for his followers. It is in man to desire to be more than man. Pride drives him to eat the apple in order to be like God, determining for himself what is good and evil. Man yearns to climb every fence, to acknowledge no limits, to leave no moon unsullied by his relentless treading. But secreted in the apple are razor blades. Each bite cuts within. Guilt festers. Seeking godlike perfection, man experiences imperfection in himself. Man is a beast of prey to man, even to the Man on the cross. Yet that Man's suffering forks lightning: a flash that brings us out of the dark. Accepting the gift of forgiveness, humanness is restored. No longer need we torture ourselves with catalogs of misdeeds. God-with-us forgives the worst that we can do to him, permitting us to forgive ourselves. Dust and spit applied by the fingers of the Healer open our eyes to the humanizing potential of suffering.

If that were all that could be said about the passion of Christ, it would not be enough. Montaigne was humanized by suffering, but his bearing of illness made no change in man's fear of the Grim Reaper. Had Jesus remained in the tomb, his words might have continued to fork lightning, but men would have gone on asking if the monkey-rope were cut at death. But Jesus didn't stay in the tomb. On the third day after burial, transformed yet bearing the marks of torture, he appeared to Mary. Therefore the early church was correct in insisting upon the supreme importance of the resurrection. Being raised from the dead, Christ raises us from the tomb of fear in which we bury ourselves. Salvation from death was the common understanding in the second and third centuries of what Christ came to give to man. Christians in that period did not follow the Greek tradition of ascribing immortality to man. They began with the Old Testament notion that man, even his soul, was mortal, subject to death. Against this view they pressed their affirmation that God gives the gift of life on the other side of death through the resurrection of Jesus Christ.

In our day the resurrection has been deemphasized because supposedly cultured debaters about religion have difficulty believing in it. Some believers have deleted from their creed any reference to Christ's "descent into hell" because they have shucked the child's ability to see the reality of the illogical. The former action deprives the one who rages against the approaching darkness of any rage-aborting hope. The latter prevents Christians from criticizing those medical practitioners who grasp at every means to snatch the dying back to life (see chapter 9).

As noted previously, in the Old Testament, hell or Sheol was the realm of the dead who were not quite extinguished. There the formerly living existed in a state of utter weakness. Going there, the monkey-rope binding them to God was cut. The childlike imagination pictured a place with bolted doors. From Adam and Eve onward, no one got out. In hell, the dead were cut off from human society and from God. What the doctrine of Christ's descent into hell was intended to proclaim was the truth that God's love reaches even to those who died before the resurrection. Although no one could be sure of it before that third day, God never cuts the monkey-rope binding man to Himself.

Albrecht Dürer made an engraving of what Christian art terms the *Harrowing of Hell* in 1512. Christ has shattered the bolted doors and is leading death's captives out of bondage, beginning with Adam and Eve whose pre-apple beauty has been recreated. Monster Death watches with alert and jealous eyes, but he is impotent. He may move men to be angry with the coming of darkness, but he cannot imprison those who commend their spirits to God. Death does not cut the monkey-rope. God dispatched his Son to the kingdom of the dead to certify that his love penetrates to the depths of despair. Man need not fight death with no holds barred.

Rightly understood, all that has been said is summarized in Jesus' question: "Which of you by taking thought can add one cubit unto his stature?" (Matthew 6:27, KJV). It is necessary to stress right understanding here. "Taking thought" has a positive connotation for us. It suggests making a budget, buying insurance, planning the use of time—all worthwhile activities. But "taking thought" meant something quite different in the early seventeenth century when the King James Version was prepared. A note in the royal court record indicates that a lady-in-waiting died because of "taking thought." She did not expire because she planned ahead. She died because she worried herself to death. "Taking thought" meant to worry oneself sick. And "stature" referred to length of life. Understanding these two terms, the meaning of the text comes clear. Jesus told his followers not to worry themselves sick about length of life. Over the number of the days of their years they had no control, except to decrease them by anxiety. Besides, *when* death comes to one is not of supreme importance, since death does not cut the monkey-rope binding man to God. "Do not worry yourself to death about dying," said Jesus, "because death has lost its capacity for intimidation."

The umbilical cord binds the fetus in the womb to his mother. A monkey-rope binds the deceased in his tomb to God. There is no need to rage against death's darkness. The tomb is a womb with a view. Nevertheless, many people persist in "taking thought" about dying. So doing, they may hasten personal and racial extinction. Their model is Kamongo.

5. SUBTILIZING OUR MINDS

Some forgotten books merit reading twice in a row. One such is Homer W. Smith's narration of the quest for the lungfish, called Kamongo[1] by the Africans. Over four hundred million years ago, this fish developed lungs, thus escaping death which stalked it in stagnant pools. Now, decreasing in numbers and nearing extinction, lungfish interest the kidney researcher and the philosopher of history.

The scientist is fascinated by the way in which Kamongo's kidneys cease to function for as long as several years while it sleeps in the mud. Lungfish normally live in lakes and rivers. However, if they are trapped in a swamp at the onset of a drought, they dig in and breathe by means of their lungs. Blanketed by hard mud, the lungfish cannot possibly eat. Kamongo therefore consumes portions of himself to stay alive. His kidneys do not function because water is lacking. Waste products accumulate in the lungfish's blood and tissues, a condition that would be fatal to other animals.

Philosophers of history reflect upon the "choice" which Kamongo made.

> This lung of his, which promised to bring him freedom from the old way of living, promised to break the bonds that chained him to a life beneath the water, but it only left him chained alternately beneath the water and the mud. If anything, he was worse off than before.[2]

By "taking thought" about survival, Kamongo chose a way

leading to death. The individual's life is lived under a sword of Damocles. Imprisoned in the mud, he eats himself to death unless water returns to set him free. If it does, Kamongo must swim forth to obtain food and elude his enemies in a weakened condition. His sleep is a tomb rather than a womb.

Kamongo is an example of specialization in the face of a changing environment. The lungfish "thought out" a means for enduring. But the means he chose is leading him along the road to extinction. Homer Smith clarifies the larger meaning of Kamongo:

> It is so common to find excessive specialization just preceding the extermination of a race that one comes to associate them together, and to accept the one as a sign of senescence presaging the other. The highly specialized animal is reaching the end of its blind alley.[3]

Man is becoming a "highly specialized animal." By "taking thought" about survival, he is inventing the technology of self-destruction. He thinks that military might will permit him to survive in the muck. Kamongo developed organs which just barely permit him to survive in the mud. Both attempts at survival may lead to extinction.

During the 1960's, the governments of the world took $1,870 billion from their peoples to buy specialized instruments for survival.[4] At least the citizens were told that their survival was being insured. In fact, the money was used by those who design, build, stockpile, and replace weapons of war. Tools of destruction have become highly specialized.

Electronic sensors were developed for use in Indochina. The movement of wind, soldiers, elephants, or children can activate them so that they send radio signals to a computer station. This "nerve center" is able to relay strike data to bombers flying over the area of activity. A pilot need not see his target, for computers will release destruction at the right time.

Kamongo devised a means for living in mud. He "took thought" about survival. Using the organs available, the lungfish entered a blind alley. "Departments of defense" are preparing more and better ways to be offensive in the dark. They are "taking thought" about survival. Perhaps they are leading mankind into a cul-de-sac. Someday water may not soften the mud of the last lungfish. Someday the last man may gape at a TV screen linked to a computer.

I suppose that even the most ardent advocates of military superiority would admit that their accomplishments could lead to human extinction. It is more difficult to see medical science as a means for "taking thought" which may be thinking us to death. After all, medicine is devoted to preserving life. Physicians dedicate themselves to that objective. And ours is a better world in which to live because of their successes. Yet those accomplishments could prove deadly to mankind. The reduction of infant mortality is speeding population growth. Babies live who once would have died. Healthier children become healthier adults who, in turn, give birth to even more healthy children. Each individual case is a blessing. Spread across the planet, however, population expansion is frightening. Even if the current downward trend in some countries were to continue, earth as a whole could discover that the life-span of the race is shortened by medicine's lengthening of individual lives.

A second problem relating to medical achievements is that because costs are high, someone must decide which sufferers are to live.

In 1971, nearly 5,000 Americans were undergoing regular kidney dialysis. Without that washing of their blood, they would have died. Lacking funds to pay for such treatments, some people do die.

A number of years ago, the Swedish Hospital in Seattle set up a committee to establish guidelines for accepting patients for kidney dialysis. The committee members approached their assignment thoughtfully. They agreed upon what they needed to know for making a decision in each individual case. These factors were enumerated:

> age and sex; marital status and number of dependents; income; net worth; emotional stability, with particular reference to the patient's capacity to accept the treatment; educational background; nature of occupation; past performance and future potential; and the names of people who could serve as references.[5]

Let us apply these factors to a specific person. He is thirty years of age, a confirmed bachelor, who lives mostly with his parents. Last year he reported a net income of $8.71½ and listed his assets as some unsold books. One reference says that "he is the most unmalleable fellow alive." Of himself he writes: "The greater part of what my neighbors call good I believe in my soul to be bad, and if I repent of anything, it is very likely to be my good behavior." Educated at Harvard, he is now employed as an "inspector of snowstorms and rainstorms." He has written a book which did not sell, but thinks only about writing another. His name: Henry David Thoreau. When David Sanders and Jesse Dukeminier, Jr., examined the criteria used by the Swedish Hospital committee, they remarked in their report that "the Pacific Northwest is no place for a Henry David Thoreau with bad kidneys."[6] Thoreau was too strange a man to be passed by such a committee. Our definitions of human worthwhileness exclude such persons. By being rejected, however, they challenge the road we have taken.

Loren Eiseley retells a story by Walter de la Mare to make this point. A traveler is reading the inscriptions on stones in a country cemetery. With the coming of darkness, he turns to leave. A stranger has suddenly come from nowhere. "The stranger, who appears to be holding a forked twig like that which diviners use, asks of our traveler, the road. 'Which,' he queries, 'is the way?'" With a movement of his arm the traveler points out the high road to town. The stranger's face expresses revulsion. Eiseley reflects that we are "suddenly tormented with the notion that our road, the road to town, the road of everyday life, has been rejected by a person of divinatory powers who sees in it some disaster not anticipated by ourselves."[7]

Just such a stranger was Henry David Thoreau. He asked the way of his neighbors in Concord. When they pointed to business as usual, he recoiled in horror. One man's life was saying: "I am a blacksmith taking thought about financial security in my old age." Another man's flesh was asserting: "I am a farmer worrying about the price of corn in Boston." Thoreau saw that they were, by "taking thought" about expiring, already breathing their last. Fretting about the future, they failed to live in the *now*. It was Thoreau's aim to make certain that he lived before he died.

Accordingly, Thoreau went off to dwell by Walden Pond. He wanted to find out what he could do without. It was his goal to simplify his life. If, he asked himself, so much seed and labor is required to make the Walden-side earth say "beans," how much seed and labor is necessary to get this flesh of mine to say "Henry David Thoreau"? The purpose of flesh is to body-forth a unique personality. If it fails to do that, it is dead. If it succeeds, it is truly alive—yet it has certain needs of its own: food, clothing, shelter. How can these needs be met without destroying one's self in the process? To answer that question, Thoreau left Concord for Walden.

What he learned is evident as Thoreau contrasts himself with his neighbor John Field. Because of his specialized needs, that Irishman became bogged down in life. Field thought that tea and coffee and butter and milk and fresh beef were necessities of the flesh. Hence, he did "bogging" for a neighboring farmer, turning up a field with a bog hoe at the rate of ten dollars an acre. Because Field worked hard, he had to eat hard to repair the damage to his flesh. It was a vicious circle in which the flesh of this laborer came nowhere near getting the essential John Field expressed. On the other hand, Thoreau simplified his needs. Eating fish instead of beef, he could sink a line into himself while holding a line to catch his dinner. Not worrying about money to buy butter and beef, he did not require coffee and tea to soothe his nerves. Because he built his own cabin, there was no rent to pay. Less income was necessary. By working as a laborer for forty or fifty days a year, he earned all he needed to keep flesh and breath of life together. The other three hundred or more days were spent cultivating a small amount of congealed dust in order to make it say "Henry David Thoreau." Along the customary road of everyday life, people get into ruts seeking unnecessary "necessities." They are wasting life on what is not required by the flesh—in fact, on what is deadly to it. Thoreau remarked that "the cost of a thing is the amount of what I will call life which is required to be exchanged for it, immediately or in the long run."

Thoreau simplified the externals of life in order to "be a Columbus to whole new continents and worlds within . . . , opening new channels, not of trade, but of thought." But such inward exploration is disconcerting. It is less upsetting to explore the outer world.

> What was the meaning of that South Sea Exploring Expedition, with all its parade and expense, but an indirect recognition of the fact that there are

continents and seas in the moral world, to which every man is an isthmus or an inlet, yet unexplored by him, but that it is easier to sail many thousand miles through cold and storm and cannibals, in a government ship, with five hundred men and boys to assist one, than it is to explore the private sea, the Atlantic and Pacific Ocean of one's being alone.8

Recently three men found it easier to fly to the moon in a government capsule, backed up by thousands on the ground, than to be Columbuses to moral seas. When astronauts James B. Irwin, Alfred M. Worden, and David R. Scott left for the moon in 1971, hidden in the pockets of their space suits were four hundred envelopes bearing stamps canceled at Cape Kennedy shortly after midnight on the day of liftoff. Carrying them for the purpose of making money violated regulations of the National Aeronautics and Space Administration. When the violation was uncovered, the astronauts said that they planned to use the money derived from selling the envelopes to set up trust funds for their children.9

There are unexplored white spots on the moral map. Technological developments make it possible to land men on the moon. So many men have now been trained to make the trip that we can no longer name them. By almost any standard, these men are well paid for their travels. Yet to gain a bit of extra money, some of them went against regulations. By "taking thought" our civilization has devised tools for a landing on the moon. We enable men to walk with heavy shoes on the ancient symbol of madness instead of exploring the islands of lunacy within.

More than one hundred years ago, Thoreau questioned this tendency. Our road of everyday life was questioned by a stranger, a man who suddenly appeared in the midst of Concord's business as usual. When he asked directions of his neighbors, their pointing dismayed him. Their lives, Thoreau saw, were ones of "quiet desperation." By "taking thought" they were dying without ever having lived. Nevertheless, those who live lives of "quiet desperation" are still those whose dying is prolonged by dialysis, if the Swedish Hospital guidelines are followed, while this world "is no place for a Henry David Thoreau with bad kidneys."

Our way has been questioned by a farsighted stranger, but we continue to walk, to drive, to soar along it. We inflate the external and deflate the internal. The English painter-poet William Blake once said: "You never know what is enough unless you know what is more than enough." Our society is dedicated to finding out what is more than enough, but the findings are not used to set standards of sufficiency. For example, architect Richard Stein quotes research indicating that three to ten footcandles provide adequate light for reading. Brighter light can be tiring. Yet when I was pastor of a church which housed a United States Government Get-Set School, inspectors demanded we provide sixty to seventy footcandles. Forty percent of America's electricity is used for lighting. Americans are willing to endure brownouts and blackouts in order to have more light than is needed at other times.[10]

Ours is a consumer economy, based not upon genuine needs but upon brain-created ones. From our minds come needs that flesh knows nothing of. We are dedicated to determining what is excessive. But our destination is suggested by W. H. Auden:

> The Road of Excess
> leads, more often than not, to
> The Slough of Despond.[11]

Russian commissars evidence some concern about that slough. They sent a display of Russian arts and crafts to the United States in 1972. Included were works of Christian art. One was a fourteenth-century icon depicting the fiery chariot of Elijah. The land of "atheistic materialism" sent works of the spirit, while America reciprocated with an exhibit entitled "Research and Development, U.S.A." On display were

> a Princess telephone, a fiberglass canoe, a Lincoln Continental, a copying machine, a computer system, a home hair dryer, a snowmobile, and an electric toothbrush. Frank Shakespeare, director of the U.S. Information Agency, said that "what we are attempting to do is reflect the fact that much of the production of the United States is oriented to the needs of the consumer. . . ."[12]

Another way of describing the situation would be to say that Western Europe and North America share a "potlatch" approach to life. A potlatch is an American Indian ceremony. Certain tribes of the Pacific Northwest stage it in order to impress their rivals. The ceremony is an exercise in boasting and consumption. A chief invites guests. To impress them, gifts are given and valuable items destroyed. Once a host killed his slaves to show how wealthy he was. During the middle of the nineteenth century, the rivalry between two tribes became so intense that they borrowed from outsiders in order to continue consuming the unnecessary. From the brain of man come needs, in the meeting of which his own bankruptcy draws near.

The late Columbia University historian Richard Hofstadter reports: "It is hard now to imagine, but it is a matter of record that a mid-eighteenth-century mariner approaching the American strand could detect the fragrance of the pine trees about 60 leagues, or 180 nautical miles, from land."[13] Two centuries later, Paul R. Ehrlich writes that "each American has roughly fifty times the negative impact on the earth's life-support systems as the average citizen of India."[14] Because dreams are not rooted in needs, the future approaches as a nightmare.

Potlatch-consumption is not going unquestioned. The young are rejecting the assertion that it is necessary to dream up needs and then to destroy what has been manufactured in order to survive as an economy. They find Francis of Assisi appealing. Over 700 years ago, he rejected the Establishment, started what has been termed the world's first youth movement, and went about Italy preaching to birds. It all began when Francesco Bernardone, son of a wealthy merchant, sold cloth from his father's warehouse and gave the proceeds to the poor. Such "ripping-off" of the Establishment makes sense to today's radicals. "Steal from the rich to give to the poor" is their motto. Their practice indicates a desire to steal from the rich in order to help the poor, while themselves living off their wealthy fathers. Thus, if they were to study the whole life of St. Francis, their admiration might wane. When the senior Bernardone discovered a shortage in his inventory, he called Francis to an accounting before the bishop in the town square of Assisi. Confronted with the facts, Francis did not deny them. He said that he must obey his heavenly Father rather than his mortal sire. Then Francis stripped to the skin, handed all his clothes back to his father, and departed to find out on his own just what was needed to sustain his life. Are today's youth sufficiently disciplined to follow Francis and Thoreau?

If not, if they are self-seeking, then no member of the Establishment dare be self-righteous. Youth have learned their selfishness and lack of discipline from their elders. They have looked at what Melvin Maddocks calls the "gold list":

> Hugh Hefner draws $303,874 out of *Playboy* magazine—more than 20 times as much as a New York detective's salary and about 10 times as much as the distinguished Oxford philosopher Sir Isaiah Berlin is paid to teach a year at City University of New York. A ballet dancer is worth $8,000 on the gold list, David Brinkley and Walter Cronkite, $250,000 each. A second-grade teacher rates $7,500. Dave De Bussschere of the New York Knicks tips in at $100,000.[15]

Selfishness is not a prerogative of the young. The pay scale of their world bears scant relationship to genuine needs.

From the mind of man come distinctions which make no sense to a Thoreau who is determined to simplify, to reduce life's needs to those which are genuine. Such a call for simplification does not, however, mean imitating "simple peoples." The inhabitants of the Ponape Islands of the South Seas are "simple" in some respects, but they also make distinctions which have no rootage in necessity. Bananas and yams are both vital to their diet. Yet for a reason not understood by outsiders, the man who owns yams is respected, while the one who harvests bananas is at the bottom of the "gold list." Such a way of calculating is simpleminded, not simple. For man to achieve true simplicity he must become subtle-minded.

Long accustomed to want, Herman Melville subtilized his mind. In *Typee* and *Omoo*, he narrated the glories of primitive humans. He saw a certain splendor in their lack of sophistication. But Melville never relaxed in the comfortable illusion that simplemindedness will restore humanness to man. He used his watches in the crow's nest to think, not to daydream. What he saw from that vantage point was a monkey-rope world.

> Yet I tell you that upon one particular voyage which I made to the Pacific, among many others we spoke thirty different ships, every one of which had had a death by a whale, some of them more than one, and three that had each lost a boat's crew. For God's sake, be economical with your lamps and candles! Not a gallon you burn, but at least one drop of man's blood was spilled for it.[16]

Here is more evidence that ours is a monkey-rope world. Every whaling-era congregation gathered for evening worship was able to read the scriptural command to be nonviolent because human blood had been shed. Lovers meeting to pledge undying love sat until the whale-oil lamp burnt out without recollecting that a life had burned out to light their tryst.

Melville's Ahab groans: "Cursed be that mortal inter-indebtedness which will not do away with ledgers."[17] Roger Shinn makes an entry in the world's books:

> The Green Revolution has achieved its amazing success in increasing food production at a cost of intensified use of fertilizers and insecticides, which when employed massively interfere with the food cycle and threaten life. The distribution of food—currently a graver problem than its production—requires a transportation net and industrial system that takes land out of agricultural use and increases pollution.[18]

Another entry is suggested by a cartoon entered in a competition at the Montreal Expo '67. Created in Czechoslovakia, it makes its comment against the background of advances in medical science made by doctors operating near fields of battle. In this sixty-second cartoon, a man on the operating table is surrounded by surgeons and nurses. When the operation is completed, the patient gets up, dresses himself in military uniform, gives a salute to the physicians, and marches off the screen. Then comes the sound of the shot that kills him.[19] War produces injuries. Those injuries draw forth new medical procedures which are of benefit to soldier and civilian alike. But the soldier is saved today only to be shot tomorrow.

We can easily become indignant about each of these instances and we make sweeping judgments. Insecticides are bad; medical advances which stem from war are bad. A good pursuit, however, may have bad consequences; and from an evil such as war come some benefits. With eyes wide open we miss "mortal inter-indebtedness." Lacking subtle minds, we see things as either good or bad.

While I was drafting this chapter, our daughter came into the room and put a picture beside my writing pad. Her chosen color was yellow. With it she sketched a house beneath the sun. Someone—probably myself—had made a charcoal fire. Another man was making an "unhappy" face at me because pollution is "bad for the birdies." In so many ways Anne is right. She got the message, with her eyes wide open, that smoke is harmful. It fouls fresh air. On the other hand, her mind is not yet sufficiently subtle to grasp the fact that civilization was made possible by the discovery of fire. Minds like hers come in adult sizes.

In *Moby Dick,* Ishmael remarks on how small are the eyes and ears of the whale in contrast with the bulk of his body. He asks:

> Is it not curious, that so vast a being as the whale should see the world through so small an eye, and hear the thunder through an ear which is smaller than a hare's? But if his eyes were broad as the lens of Herschel's great telescope; and his ears capacious as the porches of cathedrals; would that make him any longer of sight, or sharper of hearing? Not at all.—Why then do you try to "enlarge" your mind? Subtilize it.[20]

If we are to make adult ethical judgments, we must subtilize our minds. Instead of simpleminded dilation, contraction is called for. In a world where minds are dilated, actions are either black or white, good or evil. What is required is a subtle-mindedness which enables one to see that good deeds may have bad hangers-on. And from evil does come good.

Fortunately the human mind is capable of making fine distinctions. It is an instrument of generalization which, so far, has permitted man to avoid the fate of Kamongo. Homer Smith writes:

> There is the difference that sets [man] farthest apart from the other animals— his brain. There is his own unique and priceless specialty, a mass of nerve cells developed beyond any parallel in the animal kingdom! He has gone in for specializing that particular organ in preference to teeth or skin or bones.[21]

Man has specialized an instrument of generalization which allows him to be subtle-minded when he chooses to discipline his thinking.

With such a brain man can see that Kamongo's "decision" to develop a lung was both good and bad. Good, because it gave the lungfish a means for surviving changing conditions. Bad, because it appears to be leading to Kamongo's extinction. By "taking thought" Kamongo dealt with an outside death-bearer only to create in himself its replacement.

Man is able to recognize that excessive specialization often precedes the extermination of a race. His brain is capable of making such generalized judgments. It is also capable of that specialization which makes moon exploration possible and moral exploration improbable. By "taking thought" about military preparedness, man may have chosen the road to Armageddon. By "taking thought" about prolonging the lives of individuals, man may be shortening his racial life. All depends upon whether he inflates the external or deflates it, whether he specializes his mind or subtilizes it. All depends upon whether man uses his mind to distinguish in order to extinguish, or whether he uses that priceless instrument of generalization to sense the "mortal inter-indebtedness" of his monkey-rope world.

6. DISTINCTIONS AND ACTS OF EXTINCTION

A grisly item in the Metropolitan Museum's collection of musical instruments is a central African kissar. The maker of this lyre sliced off the top of a human skull, leaving a fringe of hair, and stretched a piece of skin over the brain cavity. Sticking out of the ear openings are gazelle horns which are joined by a crossbar. From this bar six strings reach back across the drum.

This kissar is doubly symbolic. It symbolizes the creative power of the human brain. From its depths come the sounds of music which go on resounding after the composer is dead. From its depths, secondly, come the distinctions which permit acts of extinction. For the Africans who made this kissar, the world is divided between those who play these lyres and those who are preyed on to obtain the skulls. The human brain accommodates those who make music and those who use their fellows to make the instruments.

Brain-created distinctions permit acts of extinction. That point is made by the history of Ireland. During the recent years of violence, one rebel priest proclaimed that they were fighting a "holy war against pagans and people who have no respect for human dignity."[1] Once the enemy is labeled as pagan and less than human, any means to his extinction is justified.

For our purposes, the first brain-created distinction in Irish history occurred in the middle of the twelfth century. An Irish king, driven off by his subjects, turned to English King Henry II for succor. Before coming to his aid, Henry asked the pope for permission. The pope, who happened to be English, granted it, and Raymond the Fat was thereupon dispatched to subdue Ireland.

During the next few centuries, England made only sporadic attempts to dominate her Irish possession. The Reformation, however, changed that laxity by emphasizing another brain-created distinction. England was Protestant; Ireland was Roman Catholic. That difference provided justification for subduing unruly subjects. At the Battle of Kinsale in 1601, the army of Queen Elizabeth I defeated the last of the great Irish earls. Later in that century, England's own deposed king, James II—a convert to Catholicism—began to raise troops in Ireland. William of Orange was dispatched. He put down the rebellion at the Battle of the Boyne. With that historic event, orange and green became colors of distinction, marking people for extinction. Catholics used Protestant violence to excuse their deeds of extinction. And Protestants used those deeds to justify their own.

Erasmus of Rotterdam noted this human inclination toward distinguishing and extinguishing. He watched Catholic fighting Protestant over distinctions concerning hell, turning Europe into a burning hell in the process. So Erasmus raised the pertinent question:

> Does not the Lord's Prayer teach concord? How can you say *Our* Father if you plunge steel into the guts of your brother? Christ compared himself to a hen: Christians behave like hawks. Christ was a shepherd of sheep: Christians tear each other like wolves.[2]

Man is a wolf to man because his brain enables him to make distinctions unknown to wolves. No wolf divides wolves into two groups: those who make kissars and those who are killed to get the raw materials. In fact, the so-called "wolfishness" of wolves owes more to the human brain's ability to project evil qualities onto others than to any actual characteristic of the unprovoked wolf.

Looking at how brain-created distinctions permit men to "plunge steel into the guts" of other men, we can only wonder if there is anything capable of clearing the brain and softening the heart of kissar-sculpting man. Is man fated—because he possesses a brain—to extinguish himself by distinctions?

Perhaps not. Occasionally a true man appears. By being what

he is, he melts the hearts of others. Such a person was Queequeg. Melville describes him as "a creature in the transition state—neither caterpillar nor butterfly." At first, Ishmael was terrified of this transitional being. He records his emotions: "Ignorance is the parent of fear, and being completely nonplussed and confounded about the stranger, I confess I was now as much afraid of him as if it was the devil himself who had thus broken into my room at the dead of night."[3] This Queequeg was a stranger, not unlike the one in Walter de la Mare's tale. He came from no place that could be pinpointed on a map. "Queequeg was a native of Kokovoko, an island far away to the West and South. It is not down in any map; true places never are."[4] He was black and tattooed. Daily Queequeg performed his devotions before a little hunchbacked ebony image. No wonder that Ishmael was terrified when this "savage" jumped into bed with him.

But proximity helps clear the mind. Ishmael began to use his brain to meditate rather than to distinguish. As he reflected, he came to see Queequeg as a fellow human being.

> For all his tattooings he was on the whole a clean, comely looking cannibal. What's all this fuss I have been making about, thought I to myself—the man's a human being just as I am: he has just as much reason to fear me, as I have to be afraid of him. Better sleep with a sober cannibal than a drunken Christian.[5]

Some time after this clearing of the brain came a melting of Ishmael's heart. A stranger revealed to him that the heavily traveled road was the inhumane one. "I felt a melting in me. No more my splintered heart and maddened hand were turned against the wolfish world. This soothing savage had redeemed it."[6] With that redemption came triumph over the world's most damnable distinction: that between black and white. White Ishmael walked arm in arm with black Queequeg. Onlookers, rutted in brain-created distinctions, "marvelled that two fellow beings should be so companionable; as though a white man were anything more dignified than a whitewashed negro."[7] Queequeg humanized Ishmael.

What this true man did for Ishmael points to the mission of the truest man of all: Jesus the Christ. It can be said of this Jesus that he was "a creature in the transition state—neither caterpillar nor butterfly." He was not crawling man, bound to dirt and the ways of man upon the earth. Neither was Jesus the winged breath of God, lacking flesh. He was *Man*. Like Adam on Michelangelo's Sistine ceiling, he was man in the flesh, but with a pulse beating in harmony with the heart of God.

One day this Man spoke. His purpose was to clear the brains of men of those distinctions which favor deeds of extinction. We call his words the Sermon on the Mount. Some interpreters view this message as being aimed at men's emotions, but that was not the original intention. Jesus sat down to speak. Greek philosophers and Jewish rabbis sat when they planned to offer reasoned discourse. Seated, Jesus attempted to alter some kissar-making brains.

For centuries men used past violent acts to justify violence in reprisal. Lamech pulled no punches: "I have slain a man for wounding me, a young man for striking me. If Cain is avenged sevenfold, truly Lamech seventy-sevenfold" (Genesis 4:23*b*-24). Lamech responded with annihilation to a nick. It did not take long for man's brain to escalate violence. When Lamech is remembered, then one customary *justification* for violence is seen as a biblical *limit* to revenge, namely, "If any harm follows, then you shall give life for life, eye for eye, tooth for tooth, hand for hand, foot for foot, burn for burn, wound for wound, stripe for stripe" (Exodus 21:23-25). To hear these words in their original context is to hear them as a prohibition of escalation. No more Lamech-like violence. If a man strikes you, strike him back; *don't* kill him. The Old Testament limited violence.

Jesus asked his followers to consider the complete transformation of violence. "You have heard that it was said, 'An eye for an eye and a tooth for a tooth.' But I say to you, Do not resist one who is evil. But if any one strikes you on the right cheek, turn to him the other also" (Matthew 5:38-39). Lamech murdered a man for striking him. Moses limited vengeance to a strike for a strike. Jesus commended the offering of more flesh to receive insulting blows.

Saul Alinsky provides a commentary on Jesus' text. As a youthful gang member, Alinsky got into a fight when he crossed over into the turf of rivals. Cops appeared, took him to the station house, and called his mother. She picked him up and escorted him to the rabbi, who lectured Saul on the wrongness of his behavior.

But I stood up for myself. I said, "They beat us up and it's the American way to fight back, just like in the Old Testament, an eye for an eye and a tooth for a tooth. So we beat the hell out of them. That's what everybody does." The rabbi just looked at me for a minute and then said very quietly, "You think you're a man because you do what everybody does. But I want to tell you something the great Rabbi Hillel said: 'Where there are no men, be thou a man.' I want you to remember it." I've never forgotten it.[8]

It may be the American way to "beat the hell out of them." But it is not the humane way.

Where there were no men, Jesus was the Man. He refused to let violence done to him serve as a justification for escalation. A village of Samaritans wouldn't receive him. James and John proposed that he call down fire from heaven to consume such stubborn men. Jesus would not hear of it. "The Son of man is not come to destroy men's lives, but to save them" (Luke 9:56, KJV). Many a Vietnamese village has had fire rained down upon it because it refused to accept a savior from Saigon or from Hanoi.

Again, when Peter wanted to use a sword to resist those who came to arrest his Master, Jesus told him to put it away (Matthew 26:52). Neither would he call upon "twelve legions of angels" to fight on his behalf (Matthew 26:53). For Jesus, being a man meant loving his enemies.

Jesus urged his followers to clear their brains of those distinctions which enable men to fashion kissars from their fellowmen. The earliest Christians gave literal adherence to this admonition to be men where there were no men. They refused to render military service within the Roman Empire.[9] But that refusal did not prevail. Before the end of the second century, Christians began serving as soldiers. Then the teachings of Jesus resurfaced. Christians were put to death in Africa, toward the close of the third century, because they refused to be drafted into the army. The position of the church became less rigid just after A.D. 300. Followers of Christ were permitted to be peacetime soldiers, but they were admonished to refuse to bear arms in time of war.

With the conversion of the Emperor Constantine to the Christian church came the conversion of Christianity to the theory of the Just War. Sometimes the reasoning began with this question: What should a Christian do if he were to happen upon the scene while that man—later treated by the good Samaritan—

was being beaten? Should he hide in the bushes only to emerge when the assailant departed? Or, should he resist the attacker even to the extent of killing him? Confronted with that question, many Christians decided that there are times when killing is justified. From that conclusion came the development of the seven conditions which must prevail simultaneously if a war is to be reckoned just: (1) The war must be fought for a good cause. (2) That goodness must not change during the fighting. (3) Before going to war, all alternatives must have been tried. (4) The methods of war must be fair. (5) It must be expected that fighting will be more beneficial than declining to fight. (6) The maker of war must be sure of victory. (7) Peace treaties must be just and must serve to prevent the outbreak of another war. In theory these conditions controlled the warring of Christians for centuries. In practice, if a state wanted to fight, it was always able to "arrange" the facts in order to make them fit the procrustean bed of Just War rationalization.

There are always those, however, who reject the justification of killing. They insist upon taking Jesus seriously. Today we call them conscientious objectors. In the Middle Ages they were often followers of Francis of Assisi who even refused to do violence to animals. Francis rejected a dreamed-of career as a soldier in order to devote his life to improving the lot of the poor. Those who came after him continued this concern for the impoverished but with a difference. They used flaming words to oppose war and to support the poor. Their language was violent.

Thomas Aquinas gave some advice to pastors. According to him, if a poor man stole, the confessor ought not to treat that action as a sin. What he took was his due. If the heart of the rich man had not been hard, there would have been no need to steal. What began in the mind of Thomas as an admonition not to make the plight of the poor worse by accusing them of sinning became in the minds of others a positive command to plunder the rich. They viewed the possession of wealth as a crime. And, while they opposed the wars of nations, they urged the plundering of the wealthy.

All of these attitudes are current. There are those who maintain that a citizen should always support his nation when it goes to war, but that individuals have no right to band together to fight exploitation. Others oppose the battles of nations, claiming the rights of conscientious objectors, but speak violently in behalf of the poor. Their fighting words result frequently in deeds of violence. This latter tendency is apparent today in discussions of the gap between the rich and the poor. In the United States the lowest fifth of families in 1967 got about 3.2 percent of the national income, while the highest fifth got 45.8 percent, fifteen times as much.[10] These figures point to a bad situation in the U.S. which continues, but the plight of the poor in the rest of the world is much worse. When these facts are comprehended, anger wells up. Sensitive people shout that something must be done. Being sensitive, these people are easily frustrated, and they move all too readily from seeing to shouting to slaying. Is killing justified if carried out on behalf of or by the impoverished?

To gain perspective, if not to answer that question, let us turn to the Bible. Deuteronomy 15:11 recognizes that "the poor will never cease out of the land." That statement does not define what is *good*, but only what *is*. Compared with some people, there will always be others who are poor. And that realistic assessment holds true whether poverty is expressed in material or intellectual or aesthetic or spiritual terms. The recent history of nations that have tried to overcome the rich-poor gap, such as Russia and China, does not refute biblical realism. The poor simply do not "cease out of the land." Nevertheless, Deuteronomy 15:11 is not an endorsement of indifference. Rather, the statement of fact stands there as a preamble to a divine injunction. "For the poor will never cease out of the land; therefore I command you, You shall open wide your hand to your brother, to the needy and to the poor, in the land."

Taken by itself that verse might seem to support the attitude of colonial Bostonians, who held to a tribal view of poor relief. They opened their hands to their "brothers." They took care of their "own" poor. But vagabonds and strangers were excluded. One proper Bostonian complained that "these confounded Irish will eat us all up."[11] That kind of distinction between "our own kind" of poor and the "other" kind might seem to be supported by the term "brother" in Deuteronomy 15:11. It is overcome, however, by Leviticus 19:10: "And thou shalt not glean thy vineyard, neither shalt thou gather every grape of thy vineyard; thou shalt leave them for the poor and stranger: I am the Lord your God" (KJV). The "stranger" is to be provided for because God is the God of strangers as well as brothers.

Jesus adds to this biblical understanding of poverty. He himself was a poor man. At his birth, his parents took advantage of an exemption permitted the poor by sacrificing two doves (Luke 2:24) instead of the usual offering, a lamb and a dove. Only the poor might substitute a dove for the lamb.[12] Since he came out of such a background, we would expect that Jesus would be especially sensitive to the distress of the poor. Yet he seemingly espoused a policy which was harder on the poor than the Old Testament. Exodus 22:26-27 shows concern for protecting the debtor against the cold of night: "If ever you take your neighbor's garment in pledge, you shall restore it to him before the sun goes down; for that is his only covering, it is his mantle for his body; in what else shall he sleep? And if he cries to me, I will hear, for I am compassionate." Against this Jesus says that, if a cruel creditor sues you for your inner garment, give him also the outer one—your protection against cold nights (Matthew 5:40). "Go unclothed rather than offer resistance" is Joachim Jeremias' paraphrase.[13]

Was the compassion characteristic of God (Exodus 22:27) lacking in Jesus? No. Jesus sought to strike a balance. The poor were not to despair. Theirs *now* "is the kingdom of God" (Luke 6:20). On the other hand, Jesus plunged the rich into despair. "You cannot serve God and mammon" (Matthew 6:24). Jesus dealt harshly with the violence of the exploiters, but he did not permit the exploited to use that violence as a justification for violence on their part. The vicious circle of violence must be broken. Nothing makes violence just.

If nothing whatsoever justifies violence, is violence ever necessary in a world where Jesus is not yet the sole ruler? That question will be examined in the next chapter. In the meantime, we have seen that the Bible provides no support for those romantics who declare that violence on behalf of the poor is glorious and just. Their symbol is the upraised, clenched fist. It is appropriate. Traditionally the hand symbolizes control. The clenched hand stands for control that *will not* be relaxed. Experience shows that those who begin by favoring violence on behalf of the oppressed end up by controlling as rigidly as the oppressors they have displaced.

Writing in the *Saturday Review,* Horace Sutton argues that Frantz Fanon,

> the prophet of violence, is also the harbinger of hope. He would redress the grievances and employ violent means to do it, but in the end he is not a nihilist. His call for reconstruction, for a re-acculturation of a liberated people, for a new and liberated life, is clear and unmistakable.[14]

It is also a delusion even though Fanon was a psychiatrist. When violence is once used for destroying an evil, it is to violence that a free rein is given. Violence produces violence: nothing more, nothing less.

There is a pertinent conversation among Sir Thomas More, his wife, daughter, and son-in-law in *A Man for All Seasons* by Robert Bolt.[15] More is urged by the members of his family to arrest a man. But this man has broken no law. Nevertheless, arrest him, they say, because he is evil. Sir Thomas replies that there is no law against being evil. Yes, there is, the law of God. Then let God arrest him! Exasperated, More's son-in-law accuses him of sophistry and says that, while they are arguing, an evil man is slipping away. Unless he has broken a law, even if he be the Devil, he is free to go, replies More. Roper cries that the Devil is being given benefit of law. Whereupon More likens laws to trees. Each country is planted thick with them. They serve as a break against the wind. If then the laws are cut down to get after the Devil, no one will be able to withstand the gale.

Justifying violence is similar to cutting down a windbreak. Through the treeless land roars a whirlwind which dashes against the rocks even those who first used violence as a means to a worthwhile end. Hence, Thomas More would protect the Devil from unlawful violence in order to spare himself the same fate. Roper can't see that. He is a man who doesn't look to the consequences. His is a brain that distinguishes in order to extinguish.

The brain, with its powers of generalization and distinction, is man's greatest gift. It permits him to write music. It also permits him to fashion kissars from the skulls of his enemies. Both of these traits are human. But the latter is inhumane while the former is humane. Brains that distinguish in order to extinguish are cold and calculating, while into a brain that has been melted by contact with a true man comes a vision of our monkey-rope world.

7. CUTTING THE MONKEY-ROPE

A pusher of drugs in *The Cop,* a French gangster film, works for the syndicate. His boss orders him to switch from supplying addicts to hooking kids. He balks. Agents of the supercrook beat him and toss his body from a balcony. Angered, his friends decide to kill the pusher's assassins. The police are also looking for the assassins. But the pusher's friends arrive first and get revenge. With that the killers of the assassins become objects of pursuit by the police. One cop fires a shot into the air to signal that he understands why they did what they did. That shot is misinterpreted. The fleeing killers of the pusher's assassins return the fire. A cop is hit fatally. His colleague decides upon vengeance. Making an arrest, he uses torture to force a confession.

This movie makes clear what Jacques Ellul calls the "law of violence." Three terms describe the working of this law.[1] The first is *continuity.* Once violence is used, as *The Cop* demonstrates, there is no getting away from it. It has continued since the time of Cain. Lamech escalated it. Violence goes on and on because it simplifies things by eliminating the need for thought. Just distinguish and extinguish.

Ellul's second term is *reciprocity.* Violence on one side calls it forth from the other. All shadings disappear. The brutality of the crooks in the film appears no worse than that of the cops, especially when we discover that the police authorities have been paid off by the supercrook. This last point is heightened by the term *sameness*. Violence is violence. It is hard to draw a line between violence that binds and violence that loosens. Violence used against enslavers turns against its users and enslaves them. As Ellul puts it, "Once we consent to use violence ourselves, we have to consent to our adversary's using it, too."[2] Even a pusher who has a soft spot in his heart for kids is not justified in complaining about being beaten. He lived by doing violence to the human brain; that violence bashed in his.

The words employed by Ellul in his book *Violence* really constitute a commentary on Jesus' word: "All who take the sword will perish by the sword" (Matthew 26:52). History has yet to disprove the Master's use of the word "all." Each nation born in violence has died in it. Centuries may pass. Individual wielders of swords may die in bed. In the end, however, the arm that waves the sword is severed by it.

Perceiving the rightness of Jesus' "all," every advocate of violence seeks to excuse his use of it in the forlorn hope that the law of violence will deign to pass him by. In a letter to *The Christian Science Monitor,* John Ell of London wrote: "In the Indian subcontinent, some have justified violence because it would, they thought, be productive of political peace in the unified Pakistan state. Others have justified violence because it would be productive of freedom for Bengal."[3] What violence *produced* is the tragedy of Bangladesh. Wherever we cut into the history of that production, we encounter violence being justified as a response to violence on the part of the opponent.

In December, 1970, elections were held in Pakistan. No party won a clear majority of seats in the national legislature, but Sheikh Mujibur's Awami League gained 151 of the 153 places allotted to East Pakistan. When the president was unable to get all factions together, he postponed convening the assembly. Violence in the east was the response to this decision from the west. West Pakistani factory managers were burned alive by East Pakistanis. The president ordered more troops into the east. These soldiers had been taught to hate Bengalis and to distinguish them as traitors and India lovers. To crush the independence movement in the east, these brainwashed soldiers sought out and extinguished students, teachers, journalists, lawyers, doctors, businessmen, and other professionals. A distinguished brain marked one for extinction. After violence had changed East Pakistan into Bangladesh with the aid of India, there was more violence in retaliation. Four young men who were accused of collaborating with the West Pakistanis were beaten and tortured to death before a cheering crowd of five thousand men, women, and children.

Violence begets violence. And violence removes most—but not quite all—doubts. An Indian Christian watched the butchery in Bangladesh and commented:

> Recently my own country, India, was at war with one of its neighboring countries [West Pakistan], and I was tempted to abandon [my] principles and to "fight the enemy" with all my heart and all my soul and all my strength. But what guarantee is there that in such a situation my action will not be guided by my misinterpretation of the demands of justice?[4]

Because there was a doubt in the speaker's mind, he refrained from making the distinctions that justify extinction. He struggled to remain humane.

Doubt concerning violence's productivity surfaces as the history of America's experience with slavery is recounted. That story begins in Africa with Arabs and Moors who were the first slave traders. They kept the whole Mediterranean basin supplied with black laborers. Their profits were made possible by the habit of black kings of enslaving war captives and criminals. These kings responded eagerly to the demand for more slaves once the New World was opened to that trade. Slave-seeking bands made war as an excuse for taking captives. These unhappy prisoners were driven to market in chains.

Whites took the black slaves over from black slavers at the coast. Doctors examined them and selected the strongest. These were branded with the company's mark and dragged into the rowboats that would take them to the ship. Once aboard, they were chained together and given less space than a corpse has in its box. Many slaves courted death. They refused to eat; so a device was invented to force open the mouth. The food was poured in through a funnel. Some survived.

Arriving in the New World, these survivors had to learn a new language and new skills. Even more vital, they had to learn how to seem to jump at the master's every whim. These masters, too, had to change. For their own peace of mind they had to see blacks as beasts. That change was easier than the one required of the slaves, who were deprived of all musical solace except their voices, separated from their families, and prevented from forming lasting sexual attachments. These deprivations soon created in the slaves some of the "beastly" qualities that the owners needed to see. They drew from their brains the distinctions which justified their feelings of superiority. Thus, when blacks gave vent to the very human desire to rebel, whites felt justified in deeds of extinction. Hector St. John de Crèvecoeur tells about the punishment of one "beast" who killed the plantation overseer. Walking through the woods on the way to dinner, he came upon the culprit suspended in a cage. Birds had attacked his body and plucked out his eyes, but the black was breathing. Later his white host explained to Crèvecoeur that "the laws of self-preservation rendered such executions necessary."[5]

By the middle of the eighteenth century, there was opposition in England to slavery. On June 22, 1772, Chief Justice Mansfield wrote a decision which held that a slave became a free man when he set foot on British soil. The slave trade was banned by an act of Parliament in 1811. A decision was reached in 1833 to abolish slavery throughout the British Empire over a six-year period. Of course, none of these actions applied to the United States since, by an act of violence, all ties to the mother country had been cut.

Thus by a Declaration of Independence which proclaimed that all men are created equal, some men had the achievement of equality postponed. What would have come to slaves in 1833 under British sovereignty, came in 1863 under American. And then only with violence. The American Revolution freed no slaves. The Constitutional Convention of 1787 was interested in slavery only as one aspect of balancing the interests of the various sections of the new nation. The invention of the cotton gin gave to slave owners a new economic lease on life.

Opposition to slavery mounted during the first six decades of the nineteenth century. Abolitionists viewed slave owners as incarnations of the Devil. They would gladly cut down every law to defeat them. Advocates of slavery were forced to defend their peculiar institution. God, they said, created man as a diversity within unity, and racial differences reveal the diversity. In the case of the black race, they argued that the differences are accentuated by Noah's curse: Because Ham stared at his father's drunken nakedness, his descendants (the black race) are doomed to be servants. Its members may be saved through belief in Christ. Nevertheless, this line of reasoning continued, even believers in Christ are not intended by the Creator to intermingle; God-given racial prejudice keeps them from doing so. Those who adhered to these beliefs therefore saw Abolitionists as incarnations of the Devil and were willing to cut down the Constitution in order to preserve slavery. All the mental equipment necessary for civil war was at hand. Brain-created distinctions marked certain men for extinction.

When the American Civil War ended, those states which had upheld slavery were in ruins. Lincoln had signed the Emancipation Proclamation. Slaves were free. The Union had been preserved. Right had triumphed. The Devil had been defeated. There was rejoicing in the North, but one Northerner, who had desired Union victory, did not shout. Herman Melville looked at the triumph and saw tragedy. In 1866, he published his visions in *Battle-Pieces and Aspects of the War*. The poems did not sell. Melville's fellow citizens were too busy enjoying their war profits to buy a book that might awaken doubts. To question is human, but the victors felt superhuman in their hour of glory.

There is a parenthesis after the first stanza of Melville's "The Conflict of Convictions" which expresses the euphoric feeling of the victors.

> *(Dismantle the fort,*
> *Cut down the fleet—*
> *Battle no more shall be!*
> *While the fields for fight in aeons to come*
> *Congeal beneath the sea.)*[6]

Those were the sentiments of Unionists who thought that violence had made an end to violence. Bloodshed, they cried, produced a world safe for pulsing blood. No more would battleships be required. But Melville looked deeper and saw further. He recognized that the winners' self-satisfied shouts of triumphant righteousness boded ill for the world's future. Melville sensed that the victory of Right was unleashing forces unrecognized by the majority.

> Power unanointed may come—
> Dominion (unsought by the free)
> And the Iron Dome,
> Stronger for stress and strain,
> Fling her huge shadow athwart the main;
> But the Founders' dream shall flee.7

The poet foresaw development of the notion that American power could do no wrong. This would lead, Melville prophesied, to dominion over others. He chose as his symbol the new iron dome of the Capitol in Washington. The original one, completed in 1819, was made of wood. Man-made iron was used for the dome finished in 1863, during the heart of the civil conflict. Melville saw that iron dome casting an ominous shadow across the earth's oceans. Instead of "fields for fight" congealing "beneath the sea," those waters would carry violence to others.

It is almost as if Melville could see the shadow of the iron dome, which is topped by a statue of Freedom, falling across the rice paddies of Vietnam. *Time's* Saigon Bureau Chief, Stanley Cloud, filled in the 1972 details of the nineteenth-century seer's prophecy:

> Viet Nam has been at blazing war for 27 years. There is hardly a person anywhere in Indochina who has not been touched directly . . . by the fighting. Mothers have lost sons and daughters. Sons have lost fathers and mothers . . . . The draft touches every young man between 18 and 35—except those who can bribe their way out. . . .
> Yet it does not end, and does not even show signs of ending. A map of Indochina in 1954, with shaded areas marking Communist control, is so remarkably similar to a map of Indochina today that one is overwhelmed by the futility of it, the unspeakable inhumanity of it. . . .8

Distinctions continue to be employed as excuses for acts of extinction.

Herman Melville wrote *Moby Dick* before the American Civil War. Therefore, we may postulate that his depiction of Captain Ahab gave him a means for understanding American history and for predicting his nation's future so accurately. Ahab defined evil: It was the white whale which had taken away his leg, as a mower cuts off grass in the field. Having defined the Devil, the captain of the *Pequod* used all the navigational skill at his command to get after him. Americans make such clearcut distinctions to justify attempts at extinction. Some things are evil. They embody the Devil. They must be destroyed and, in their destruction, Right triumphs. The Devil has worn the masks of slavery, secession, facism, and communism. But whatever the mask, the means are the same. Unconditional surrender is demanded.

That Ahab-like attitude carries with it the seeds of tragedy. In a tragedy the central figure is a great man or a great nation. Nothing is commonplace about the tragic hero. His powers are extraordinary, and he throws them all into the fight against whatever threatens him. But, when the hero acknowledges no limits to his pursuit, when he demands unconditional surrender, doom hangs over him. Ahab spared no one. He went after the white whale with a harpoon whose steel point had been tempered in human blood. Violence, as we have seen, is reciprocal. Ahab hurled that blood-bathed harpoon at Moby Dick. It pierced and held, but the whale dove. The attached rope flew out of the boat so fast that Ahab was caught in its loops and carried to his extinction.

Ours is a monkey-rope world. Penguins in Antarctica suffer because Arizona farmers spray their fields with DDT. The transportation system needed for the distribution of food takes land required for its production. Medical discoveries which save individual lives may threaten human survival. Our actions drag along others. Ahab's single-minded quest of Moby Dick brought destruction to his ship, his crew, and himself. And the white whale swam on.

The message of a tragedy like *Moby Dick* is not comforting. We are not soothed in our simpleminded distinctions between good and evil. We are not confirmed in our belief that all hindrances to getting after Wrong must be leveled. We are not supported in the notion that we can passionately pursue Right without becoming entangled in evil consequences. Ours is a monkey-rope world. The good that we do may be productive of an evil that we did not will. To recognize these connections requires a subtlety of mind that shuns black-white distinctions in favor of seeing human beings. The man who looks at another man and sees a potential kissar has dilated eyes. The man who notes that skull-hunting expeditions lead to revenge is beginning to grasp the law of the sword. The man who knows that his own life is diminished when another man dies is a citizen of the monkey-rope world.

Let us return now to that section of *Moby Dick* with which we began. The basic question was whether or not Ishmael might cut the monkey-rope in order to save his own life. If Queequeg were careless and slipped into the jaws of a shark, must Ishmael follow him? According to the rules of the *Pequod,* he must. He would not be permitted to cut the monkey-rope. This narrative prepares us for dealing with what is at stake when killing is being considered or when it is a matter of letting someone die.

Suppose I come upon the scene as a person is drowning. Living in a monkey-rope world, his life is tied to mine. I offer him a chance to survive. But the day is cold. The water is swift. I am not a strong swimmer. In addition, ties of love bind me to wife, children, and others I have been ordained to serve. What shall I do? Whatever choice I make, some monkey-rope will be cut. There are those who say that the "most loving thing" for me to do is to cut the monkey-rope binding me to the drowning man in order to keep intact the network with my family and parishioners. Later we shall deal with calling such cutting the "most loving" action. It is sufficient here to note that doing the right thing in relation to one set of neighbors can leave others in the lurch. The tragic dimension is never far beneath the surface of life.

To continue our explorations in the moral world, let us imagine that we walked down the road ahead of the good Samaritan and came upon the wounded man while his assailant was at hand. Should we stand by, wait for the thug to go, and then bind up the wounds? Or should we resist that assailant with all our might, even to the point of killing him? Some argue that the "most loving" action is to cut the monkey-rope binding us to the victimizer in order to fulfill the implications of the one binding us to his victim. Whether or not such a decision is the "most loving" one remains to be determined. What is clear is that killing in defense of another involves both of us in a tragedy. One man lives because another dies, and the defender of the defenseless made it impossible for one warped human being to become straight.

Such examples as the foregoing are at the heart of an ethic that directs attention to particular situations. And situations do alter responses, as the Hebrew wisdom writer knew. He places two maxims back to back: "Answer not a fool according to his folly, lest thou also be like unto him. Answer a fool according to his folly, lest he be wise in his own conceit" (Proverbs 26:4-5, KJV). It all depends upon circumstances. Replying to some fools only entangles the respondent in their nonsense. Not replying to some fools only confirms them in their delusions. Sensitivity to all circumstances is essential.

Ought one never to tell a lie? The commandment is precise. Yet situations vary. Benjamin Constant put the pertinent question in 1797: "Would it be a crime to lie to a murderer who asks about a friend whom he wants to kill and who has taken refuge in my home?"[9] The German philosopher Immanuel Kant said it would be wrong. He believed in strict adherence to the principle of never lying. I suspect that we feel in our *reins* that Kant was mistaken. Better to tell a lie and preserve the monkey-rope binding us to the one hidden in our home than to tell the truth, thus severing the cord. Our feelings often do guide us rightly. Experience develops within us a feel for the time when it is necessary to put aside a rule. As a pastor I have learned to pay attention to sensations of uneasiness. Frequently they reveal concealed but active ingredients in a situation.

Nevertheless, an ethic which focuses upon feelings of what is right and wrong in each situation is not acceptable. Man's power of rationalization is highly developed. We can always convince ourselves that what we feel like doing is the "most loving" thing to do. Reflect upon the following account:

> The members of [a student] commune decided to abandon rules and live as they felt like living in all their activities, including sexual relations. However, it soon turned out that none of the males felt much like sharing his bed with two homely girls. The girls protested that affections were not being justly distributed and that the community owed them better. The community agreed, and set up rules by which the girls received their fair shares of the available resources.[10]

Two difficulties with situationalism surface in that account. First off, people who follow their feelings tend to ignore the feelings of others. What is *felt* to be "good" or "most loving" soon appears as sheer caprice. Monkey-ropes go unnoticed because their presence is detected by subtle minds, not dilated emotions. And, secondly, those who have been cut off tend to protest in the name of justice. They demand their due. They seek a rational ordering of affairs in which the tugging of each monkey-rope is measured.

Such protests in the name of justice bring us to a second approach to decision making. The initial assumption here is that there are similarities among situations. From a study of what is common to many cases it is possible to draw out guidelines or rules for governing choices to be made. Experience shows that the application of certain principles does achieve a balancing of interests. Melville gives an instance in *Moby Dick*. What do you do when a harpooned whale comes up under the boat which snagged him? Years of sailing on whaling ships gave shape to the guideline: "*Stick to the boat.*" If not shattered by the impact, it will right itself. If broken into pieces, you will be handy to something to cling to until rescued. On the other hand, if a novice follows his feelings and jumps, he is more likely to be killed. Now suppose that two of the ship's boats are shattered simultaneously but quite some distance apart. In the direction of which boat does the ship's officer set his course? "When placed between jeopardized but divided boats, always pick up the majority first." When you have to cut the monkey-rope, cut the one attached to the lesser number of sailors. That rule would restrain a captain whose feelings rushed toward the smaller boat that contained his son.

After reflecting upon many wars, Cicero formulated guidelines for deciding whether or not a particular military action might be termed "just." He said that the object of such killing must be the vindication of justice and the restoration of peace. Only the state can wage a "just war," and only after making a formal declaration of intent. Treaties are to be respected. Innocent persons must not be harmed. Humane treatment of prisoners is required. As we have seen, Christian leaders expanded this classic formulation and spelled out seven conditions of a "just war." That did not bring an end to reflection, however. Erasmus subjected the question to careful analysis. He saw that the theory of a "just war" rests upon the assumption that there is a similarity between warfare and the administration of justice in the state. Judges weigh the merits of both sides and decide where to strike a balance. No such machinery exists on the international scene. A nation deciding to fight judges the justice of its own cause. Since nations are no less prone to rationalization than individuals, it cannot be expected that they will apply with impartiality the seven rules for a "just war" to themselves. As a consequence, Erasmus noted that, in the absence of a truly objective international tribunal, there is no way of adjudging a war "just." And he went on to say that, in disputes over territory, justice is impossible. Every piece of land has belonged at some time to another people. How far back do you go to determine property rights in the Middle East? Erasmus' own example was that Romans have a claim to England, Spain, and parts of Africa on the basis of past occupation. Would that render an Italian campaign today against any of those lands "just"? Hardly. How then do we know that warring closer to us is less susceptible to self-deception?[11]

Modern warfare makes a mockery of the condition that the innocent must be spared. Speaking about fighting in Vietnam, General Williamson said: "We are making unusual efforts to avoid having the American young man stand toe-to-toe, eyeball-to-eyeball or even rifle-to-rifle against an enemy...."[12] A refugee reported on the success of these "unusual efforts": "One friend of mine went to the village to get rice for his mother and father to eat. He crossed the field to the hill and the airplanes saw him and shot him and killed him so that you couldn't even see his body. It was scattered all over the field."[13] If protection of the innocent is a necessary condition of a "just war," then no war in recent time—if ever—has been just.

With a glint in his sober eye, Erasmus pointed to another irrational aspect of war, namely, the cost in money. He chose the instance of Cardinal Wolsey's campaign against the French city of Tournai. Forty thousand knocked-down wooden huts were provided to house the troops during the siege. However, the French surrendered immediately. The English army returned home. And the huts served as summer houses for the citizens of Tournai. Craig Karpel has done some calculating in relation to the war in Vietnam: "We're spending approximately $133,333 for each Cong we kill, or enough to set each one up with a regional franchise for McDonald's over here."[14] The results of fighting don't appear to "justify" the expenditures of money, not to mention lives.

I began this section of my argument by suggesting that the theory of the "just war" is an example of extracting rules for action from reflecting upon similarities among situations. However, prolonged reflection has revealed that no war is, in fact, "just." Not only is there no impartial court for determining justice, but also the innocent cannot be protected and costs cannot be maintained in proportion to benefits gained. What we have discovered is this: Hard thinking about justice ought to make us chary of claiming that a particular action is "just."

That discovery brings us to Jesus' objection to the ways of the Pharisees. They cut monkey-ropes and felt justified in doing so. The injunction to support one's parents financially could be set aside by telling them that the money had been offered to God (Matthew 15:5). Jesus objected. The Pharisees had developed guidelines that permitted them to cut monkey-ropes with a clear conscience. They felt that their adherence to rules proved them "just." Such self-righteousness angered Jesus.

Complacency is the problem at the core of an ethic that permits one to say that cutting the monkey-rope can be the "just" thing to do. Complacency—if not also mendacity—clings to the assertion that cutting the monkey-rope can be the "most loving" thing to do. In each case, the person with the scissors is shielded from a view of the tragic dimension of life. Because such words as "right" and "just" and "loving" tend to suggest that the doer of the deed may have a clear conscience, I prefer to speak about that which is *exigent*. Exigency refers to absolute necessity. It may be absolutely necessary for me to let a man drown, but that exigency opens up before me a vision of my involvement in what Ahab termed "that mortal inter-indebtedness which will not do away with ledgers." I must not enter "just" or "most loving" on the credit side to balance the debit. Cutting the monkey-rope is never a "just" or "most loving" action. It may, however, be absolutely necessary. Such necessity is determined by combining the best insights of the two approaches we have considered.

As a general rule, honesty is the best policy. Long experience with situations shows that one lie sets fire to another until the liar is burned in the conflagration. Nine times out of ten, it is preferable to be candid. On the tenth occasion it is necessary to lie, to cut the monkey-rope of integrity which ties man to man. That situation is the one presupposed in Benjamin Constant's inquiry: "Would it be a crime to lie to a murderer who asks about a friend whom he wants to kill and who has taken refuge in my home?" We *feel* the answer to be no, and surely we have identified necessity. Nevertheless, this identification of exigency comes only as a result of hard thinking about guidelines. To jump to an assertion of what "the situation demands" without first considering the red flags thrown up by evaluations of similar situations is to be simpleminded. It is also to be less than humane, for humanity inheres in the habit of doubting, of subtilizing one's mind.

Exigency in terms of cutting the monkey-rope will be examined in the next two chapters in relation to the issues of abortion and euthanasia. For now, I will quote a statement from the theological encyclopedia *Sacramentum Mundi,* which summarizes my position:

> Since man's right to life is not given him by man, and man has the duty of placing himself as fully as possible in the service of life, the killing of men when forced to defend oneself can only be done within the limits of the absolutely necessary, that is, insofar as it serves the optimum preservation of life. Hence even a defensive war is unjust where the protection of the lives of the attacked is out of all proportion to the destruction let loose by the war. For the same reason, passive resistance is to be preferred in the first place to violent revolution. But even revolution may be permissible when it is the means of averting a worse reign of terror.[15]

Necessity is to be qualified with the adjective "tragic." It was necessary to save the American Union and to abolish slavery. Yet that exigency included elements of tragedy. Melville could write prophetically of the shadow of the iron dome because he had wrestled with the character of Ahab in *Moby Dick.* The situation called for Ahab to pursue Moby Dick. That whale had severed his leg, and there seemed to be something consciously malign about the bite. For Ahab the white whale embodied evil, just as slavery did for the Abolitionist. To get after the Devil, Ahab used every rule known to whaling captains. He used the accumulated experience of whalers, represented by charts of the best cruising lanes. Only at one point did he go against the guidelines. He himself went out in the boat to harpoon Moby

Dick. "Among whale-wise people it has often been argued whether, considering the paramount importance of his life to the success of the voyage, it is right for a whaling captain to jeopardize that life in the active perils of the chase."[16] Not only the breaking of a specific rule, but also his unconditional surrender attitude cost Ahab his life and the lives of all crewmen save Ishmael. The necessity to which he yielded was tragic.

Such a possibility must be reckoned with whenever we assert the necessity of cutting a monkey-rope. It was exigent to fight the Civil War, but victory bred in the victors a sense of being divinely favored. And that self-righteousness led to what Melville called the pursuit of "Power unanointed" and "Dominion." This vision of tragic consequences flowing from necessary actions —doubt about the "justice" of one's decisions—keeps us from playing Ahab.

8. ABORTION

Three of the themes woven into this book help us to evaluate America's pro-abortion climate, which is typified by the recent Supreme Court decision removing many of the legal sanctions against abortion. Of these the first is the assertion that man is a flesh-spirit unity. There is a monkey-rope linking breath of life and flesh. When one slips, the other slides. The second theme is the emphasis on determining which of man's needs are brain-created and which are inherent. His mind lifts man above the other creatures. It also permits him to pursue that which is self-destructive.

The tendency to look at life with dilated eyes constitutes the third theme. The open-eyed person sees no crossroads at which good and evil meet. Never do they travel together. The subtle-minded person recognizes that the pursuit of good can be productive of evil and that evil deeds can have good consequences. His vision is corrected by a sense of tragedy.

Cutting the flesh-spirit monkey-rope, stressing brain-created needs, and dilating the eyes: These distortions characterize many of the arguments in support of abortion on demand. Such support is mounting. In 1968, 85 percent of Americans opposed modifying legal restrictions on performing abortions. Four years later, half of all adults favored elimination of all limitations. An additional 41 percent would permit abortions under some conditions.[1] Let us see how the three distortions mentioned contribute to this pro-abortion climate.

First of all, flesh is puffed. It is said to be good. Man is urged to accept gratefully his fleshliness. It is not shameful. With these assertions of the goodness of flesh the person steeped in the Bible has no quarrel. But he is startled by the ghost met at the next turning. The disembodied spirit is held to be the essence of man. According to the popular view, man *has* flesh, but man *is* not flesh. Inner man is not tied by a monkey-rope to outer man. The ghost does not slide when the flesh slips. Essential man is inside the flesh, above it, not fundamentally bound to it. Therefore, if the ghost in the flesh does not like the consequences of fleshly acts, he feels free to repudiate them.

Abortion is favored by those, among others, who do not feel bound to their sexual acts. Sex is fun. Pleasure is stressed by those who assert that enjoyment carries with it no commitments. The Bible demurs. Man *is* flesh. Breath of life becomes visible through it. In sexual intercourse self is expressed. The invisible is made visible, and what is seen is what the man *is*. Breath of life and flesh are linked by a monkey-rope. Flesh plunging into flesh draws along the spirit. This affirmation is denied by those who try to sever flesh and spirit. They ignore the monkey-rope. Sex is a game which does not commit the inner man. He is not tied to the outcome of coitus. If conception occurs, the embryo is felt to exist in no essential relationship to the ghost in the flesh that created it. Therefore, an abortion is a means for dealing with what Natalie Shainess calls "an unfelicitous happenstance."[2]

This popular exaltation of flesh severs it from breath of life. What flesh does is not necessarily an expression of spirit. Conception indicates only that fleshly intercourse has taken place. It brings to light nothing fundamental concerning the man and woman. The thesis of George Santayana is denied:

> A child, half mystery and half plaything, comes to show us what we have done and to make its consequences perpetual. We see that by indulging our inclinations we have woven about us a net from which we cannot escape: our choices, bearing fruit, begin to manifest our destiny.[3]

Where the cord binding spirit and flesh is cut, abortion cuts loose the conceptus.

Once the inner man is separated from the outer, the brain-created needs will bear little relationship to the exigencies of the flesh. Hence, our second distortion is associated with the first. A person who feels no sense of responsibility for his acts in the flesh will find brain-created needs to "justify" his repudiation of their consequences. If sex is basically for fun, then it is on a par with other pleasures such as travel. Since both are equally needful, if conception threatens the travel budget, the fetus is aborted.

We have noted the thoughtful manner in which Thoreau calculated the exigencies of the flesh. He saw that his body required food, clothing, and shelter. No one disagreed. Thoreau's Concord neighbors said they labored to provide shelter, clothing, and food for their families. It was in his determination to provide for his fleshly needs without spending too much of life that Thoreau differed from them. John Field thought he needed roast beef. Earning money to buy it, that Irishman expended more energy than the beef restored. In the opinion of Thoreau, therefore, costly beef was a brain-created need, the pursuit of which was detrimental.

Using the categories of food, clothing, shelter, and tuition, experts working for the Presidential Commission on Population Growth and the American Future calculated the cost of a child. To rear him from birth through four years of college demands a direct outlay of $20,000. If we add to that figure the money that the mother is unable to earn while raising her family, the total comes to $60,000.[4] Since it is not unusual for four years of college alone to cost $20,000, the actual sum may be much greater than the estimate in individual cases. If these figures reflect the cost of a child, how do we measure his value?

A Michigan court of appeals faced that question. Suit was brought against a druggist by a married couple. Instead of giving the wife birth control pills which had been prescribed, the druggist gave her a tranquilizer. Calmly she conceived, but she did not want another child. The court ruled that if the couple can prove negligence on the part of the pharmacist, he must pay damages. These are to be computed by subtracting the joys of parenthood from the cost of raising a child.[5] Since the "joys" are to be subtracted from the "costs," it would seem that the court assumed that a child is worth less than other items the same amount of money could buy.

That assumption is becoming more and more popular, in part because "needs" are not scrutinized. Does a child truly need the types of food, clothing, and shelter now being purchased? Is a $20,000 college education a genuine need or a brain-created one? If the coming of a child would rule out a trip to Europe, does the need for adventure weigh heavier than the claims of living flesh?

As a society we are failing to back brain-created needs into a corner for questioning. Consequently they are permitted to "justify" actions which may be self-destructive. John Field thought he needed roast beef. To get it, he undermined his health. Such a danger may lurk in the future of all who refuse to differentiate between brain-created needs and the exigencies of the flesh.

That refusal avails itself of the services of our third distortion: dilation. Dilated minds tend, in dealing with abortion, to equate good with safety and evil with bungling. If statistics show that there are few deleterious aftereffects of a particular method, then abortion is good. The suction technique is used for most abortions during the first three months of pregnancy. A vacuum draws the dismembered fetus out through a tube into a bottle. It is claimed that the mortality risk faced by the mother is less than that encountered in giving birth. Abortions performed during months four through six are three to four times more risky.[6] Therefore, it is argued, good is an early abortion; evil is a later one.

Of course, no proponent of abortion has made such a bald equation of medical safety and goodness. Yet that dilation of the moral sense which permits it is present. The mental state is that of the film character who said that the Vietnam war was good so long as there was a possibility of victory. When that possibility faded, the war became evil. Good is equated with success and evil with failure. What is neglected is that subtlety of vision which sees that an evil pursued with good motives can fight back, turning the pursuit itself into a disaster. Ahab chased Moby Dick because he saw him as a mortal threat. When he punctured that threat with his harpoon, Ahab died; the quest proved fatal in an unexpected way. An abortion which destroys one threat to happiness may pose another. Or it may be an evil deed which is productive of some good. Never is it an unadulterated "just" act. Never is it the "most loving" thing to do. Always it does involve the participants in life's tragic dimension.

Having examined three distortions of the point of view expounded in this book, let us turn to a restatement of the basic position. Man *is* flesh. Apart from it there is no human life. Just as the foot cannot say to the hand, "I have no need of you"; so the breath of life cannot say to the flesh, "I can get along without you." Flesh makes it possible for the spirit to exercise mastery. Through the flesh the world's colors, smells, and noises are conveyed to the spirit. How the spirit reacts to these is shown by contractions of the facial muscles, movements of the hands, and words poured forth over the tongue. Breath of life is linked by a monkey-rope to the flesh. When that cord is cut, death occurs. Prior to death, what the partner at one end of the rope does involves the other. There is no slipping of the flesh which does not reveal a sliding of the spirit.

Without flesh, then, there is no human life. Where there is flesh that has the potential for giving expression to the breath of life, there is flesh that must be reverenced. Our problem is one of deciding when such flesh is present. Concerning abortion, our specific question is: At what point on the chart of fetal development, described in chapter 3, does flesh which has the possibility of making spirit visible come into existence?

What is formed at conception is unique, a never-to-be-repeated combination of genes. Unless twins develop at the point of segmentation, only one individual will ever possess this grouping of hereditary traits. Statistical evidence gives additional importance to this moment. If a sperm is destroyed, what is lost is that which had one chance in two hundred million of fertilizing an ovum. But if a zygote is destroyed, what is lost is that which had a better than 80 percent chance of bodying-forth personality.[7]

My contention is, therefore, that from conception onward we have life to which we are bound by a monkey-rope. Naturally there are those who disagree. Some feel that weeks eight to twelve constitute a vital divide. Others point to the age of viability. Many find that we are bound to a child only after birth when he becomes human through relationships. Among the Ainu, it is believed that the mother gives the child its body during pregnancy, but the soul is implanted by the father during the first twelve days after birth.[8] Electroencephalographic readings indicate that the brain becomes fully active about age one when the child begins to talk.[9]

Without question, these post-conception divides are important. Stressing one or another of them, however, permits one to extinguish life with a clear conscience. If the distinguishing divide between prehuman and human is fixed at birth, a fetus can be blithely aborted. The situation is not too different from that which prevailed during the seventeenth and eighteenth centuries in France. Animals were likened to clocks. When tortured, the noises they made were said to come from touching little springs. By definition dogs could be beaten: they were "soulless automata," feeling no pain.[10] In similar fashion, a distinction between prehuman and human can lead to heartless abortions.

On the other hand, if we maintain that there is flesh with the potential for expressing spirit from conception onward, then any cutting of the monkey-rope (abortion) must be approached with reverent caution. That caution is informed by two of this book's themes.

First of all, we must be wary of permitting brain-created needs to establish necessity for an abortion. Is the alleged need rooted in the flesh? If it is not an exigency inherent in man, it must be viewed with suspicion. On February 22, 1972, the Washington *Post* carried this banner on the sports page: "Abortion Made Possible Mrs. King's Top Year." The accompanying story reported that without an abortion Billie Jean King could not have earned $100,000 playing tennis in 1971.[11] Is such an income essential? Does the thrill of winning weigh more heavily than flesh with the potential for expressing personality? Caution demands that brain-created needs be separated from genuine ones.

Secondly, subtle-mindedness characterizes the cautious person. He knows that good and evil never travel by themselves. A pregnancy may be so bad that the monkey-rope binding the fetus to its mother must be cut. The relief experienced by the woman is good; perhaps her health, even her life, has been saved. Yet that good may cast a dark shadow.

At the graveside, a widow asked me to call upon her at home. When I did so, she seemed anxious to tell me what had happened to her forty years earlier. She and her husband desired a child. They were delighted when she became pregnant. Then complications developed and she was rushed to surgery. While she was unconscious, the doctor told her husband that there was a choice between the life of the baby and that of the mother. An abortion was performed. This woman who poured out her story to me had been spared. It was good to have had so many happy years with her husband, and yet even after all these years there was a shadow cast by the necessary destruction of the flesh that might have embodied their love.

Necessity and tragedy are companions. Because they walk together, I prefer not to say that an abortion is "just" or that it is the "most loving" thing to do. Even when it is absolutely necessary, an abortion will have varied consequences. These are similar to the scarlet letter in Hawthorne's novel. Some are worn on the outside like the embroidered *A* on Hester's dress. Some fester within and burn their way outward through the flesh like the *A* on Dimmesdale's chest.

In the book *Dialogue in Medicine and Theology,* Doctors Litin and Rynearson discuss the case of a young married woman who came seeking an abortion.[12] Her husband was overseas; the father of her child wasn't. She told the physicians that her husband was a wonderful man but that he wouldn't understand. If the doctors would not agree to an abortion, she would kill herself. Her request was granted. Some months later she wrote to say that she and her husband were happily reunited. An abortion had solved her problem.

As the doctors describe it, that case appears to be free from tragic overtones. But, since I have advised caution, let us back it into a corner. Doctor Rynearson admits that most people do not carry out suicide threats, but he felt this intelligent woman was capable of doing so. His feeling may have been correct, but statistics do not support him. Between 1938 and 1958, 13,500 Swedish women were refused abortions. Of these only three committed suicide.[13] Surely there were some intelligent and determined women among the 13,497 whose requests were not granted but who did not kill themselves. How did Doctor Rynearson know "perfectly well that the only way to save her life was to help her have a therapeutic abortion"? He didn't know; he *felt*. As we have seen, there are times when our *reins* advise us well, but only when we have exhausted the guidance which comes from comparing similarities among situations. Statistics suggest that Doctor Rynearson may have been hasty.

In the second place, Doctor Rynearson played along with the notion that a husband does not *know* about those actions of his wife which are not thrust into his line of vision. The young wife believed that what she had done in the flesh would not affect the covenant made between her and her husband if he were not told about it, if he never saw the child. Such a view of marriage is naïve. It separates flesh from the breath of life. Just as tradition holds that vows without intercourse do not constitute a marriage, so is it true that coitus outside of covenant frays the monkey-rope. The wife in this case may have thought that what her husband did not know would not hurt him, but she was mistaken. What happened to her had changed her. The monkey-rope of fleshly involvements now tied her to two men. When her husband returned, he might not learn the facts, but he would sense himself entwined in the ropes. A marriage "saved" by mendacity and abortion constitutes a house divided against itself.

Unwittingly perhaps, Doctor Rynearson helped to foster a view of man which no knowledgeable physician accepts. Surely he is aware of all that is implied when the word *psychosomatic* is used. Illness of the flesh troubles the spirit. Spiritual troubles affect the flesh. They are bound by a monkey-rope. Yet the doctor went along with a non-psychosomatic view of marriage, namely, that the behavior of the flesh is without effect on the breath of life.

Finally, it should not surprise us to learn that Doctors Rynearson and Litin resent guidelines. The latter is emphatic:

> I'm not the least bit interested in statistics. I'm not interested in how many girls commit suicide as a result of the fact that they are pregnant and could not obtain an abortion. I'm much more interested in this individual girl sitting in my office at the time. I don't want to be bound by specific or general rules. . . .[14]

His concern is to spare the person at hand some unhappiness.

In evaluating the ideas of Doctors Litin and Rynearson, some attention ought to be given to their assertion that each situation is so different from every other situation that it is impossible to generalize. They may suppose this to be true, but they could not practice medicine if it were true. That practice rests upon the assumption that patients and diseases are similar from case to case. Diagnosis depends upon similarities. No patient wants a surgeon who thinks that each cancer is so different from every other cancer that he is forced to decide in the light of each sufferer's agony what will best relieve it. Training and experience prepare the physician for the possibility that he may have to increase the patient's unhappiness in order to accomplish what a comparison with similar cases shows to be best in the long run. Something like that also prevails in ethics. Guidelines keep us from allowing emotion to sway judgment. Unfortunately, when Doctors Rynearson and Litin move from medicine to ethics, they leave behind their trained minds and yield to a situationalism that is as shapeless as the word *happiness*.

This case should make clear that caution is vital. But, where guidelines are rejected, caution evaporates. We do not need rules that predetermine our response to each request for an abortion, but guidelines which slow us down and oblige us to consider as many factors as possible.

In Deuteronomy 22:23-27, a guideline is recorded which deals with the treatment of a betrothed virgin who has intercourse with another man. If the act took place in the country, only the man is to be put to death. If in a settled area, both are to die. What is the rationale? Let us begin with what is common to all cases. The monkey-rope binding the woman to her fiancé has been cut. What can differ? Whether or not the woman called for help. If intercourse occurred in the country, no one could hear her cry, so she is granted the possibility of rape. If the occurrence was in a town, on the other hand, it is assumed that she was a willing partner since no one heard her scream.

What now is common to every case in which an abortion is sought? First of all, the pregnancy is the outcome of an act in which personalities were expressed in and through the flesh. Much more is involved than a mere rubbing of the flesh from which the spirits of the partners stand aloof. Secondly, adhering to the program which was established at the moment of conception, the zygote has a better than 80 percent chance of developing into a fetus that will be born. In the third place, this zygote or embryo or fetus does not *belong* to the mother. From both the father and the mother come the traits which, combining, constitute its uniqueness. The umbilical cord is thrown out by the new being: it is not offered by the mother. The child she carries belongs not to her, but to the stream of human life.

What can vary from case to case, thus establishing the necessity for an abortion? First, the personality embodied in the flesh of the impregnator may be so perverted as to call what is conceived into question. What I have in mind is rape where the woman is a totally unwilling partner, or incest where the risk of fetal deformity is high. In one study of eighteen incestuous pregnancies, only seven of the children were normal.[15]

Where true rape has occurred, it may be deemed necessary to cut the monkey-rope binding the woman to a child, conceived under duress and in horror and which, if allowed to live, would be the innocent object of hatred. The best procedure is to carry out a thorough uterine scraping about seven to ten days after the attack. The problem is one of establishing the woman's "unwillingness." One study of 668 complaints in the District of Columbia found that only 322 women were "victims."[16] However, these findings are open to question. Women allege police bias which makes them reluctant to report rape and uncertain of a fair hearing if they make the attempt. Understandably, then, abortions performed for rape are infrequent. In Britain during 1969, only eighty out of 54,000 abortions were attributed to that reason.[17]

Perhaps the human conditions in which incest occurs are even more perverted than those pertaining to rape. A daughter impregnated by her father may never recover from the wound to her spirit. If we need proof that flesh is tied to breath of life, then it is only necessary to look at girls who were unable to make a successful marriage due to an early incestuous relationship.[18]

Where the spirit embodied in the flesh is mad or malicious, an abortion would seem necessary. Even there, however, the Bible does not permit a callous attitude toward the embryo in the light of God's love for the outcast, the stranger.

In the second place, the fetus may pose a threat to the mother's life. Where the embryo is not growing in the uterus but rather in the Fallopian tube—ectopic pregnancy—an operation is necessary to save the mother; in reality, the pregnancy is self-terminating. The fetus will be destroyed in either case. What the operation does is to save the life of the mother. Heart and kidney failure may be fatal to a woman unless pregnancy is terminated. The prognosis in some cancer cases is better if an abortion is performed.

All of these instances are so rare, however, that one authority can say that "the life of the mother is almost never jeopardized by pregnancy."[19] Where there is jeopardy, something similar to the whaling guideline of saving the stricken boat containing the larger number of sailors applies. The doctor saves the mother who is already bound to many lives by monkey-ropes, instead of the child who has attached itself to her. But such decisions are not without shadows of tragedy. We have noted the instance of the widow who was still lamenting a lifesaving abortion performed forty years earlier.

Third, the mother's health, but not her life, may be threatened. Medical advances make it possible for many diseased mothers to survive harrowing pregnancies. They can be kept flat on their backs to ensure safe delivery. But what about the years of care? A heart that is able to endure pregnancy because of bed rest may be unable to cope with the nearly daily crises in a young child's life. The question to be considered is not only whether the woman is strong enough to carry the child for nine months, but also whether she is strong enough to carry the responsibilities for eighteen years.

In weighing that question, we must also consider the known consequences of abortion. Doctor R. F. R. Gardner writes:

> I think it would be widely accepted that abortion performed in good hands in good circumstances, within the first eight weeks from the last menstrual period, is not attended by any short-term or long-term *physical* complications in the vast majority of cases.[20]

After eight weeks the risks increase. Also, the phrase "vast majority of cases" hides the fact that, in Britain in 1969, the death rate from abortion was one-and-a-half times as high as the maternal mortality rate.[21] It is likewise true that, after repeated legal abortions, pregnancies are twice as likely to have serious complications.[22] These statistics do not take into consideration *psychological* problems and the impact on a child who learns that mother has been in the hospital to have his baby brother or sister taken away. Physically necessary and safe abortions are not immune from tragic outcomes.

The fourth variable is psychology. Just as there may be psychological reasons for pregnancy (for example, the need to establish identity through proving ability to conceive), so there may be psychological indications for abortion. Is this woman mentally stable enough to raise a child? Such a query is simple only in statement. In fact, there may be physical reasons why an abortion must not be performed, even though the woman is desperately depressed by her pregnancy. Her medical condition may be so precarious that no competent gynecologist would risk operating. There may also be psychological reasons why the psychological indication ought not be accepted. Studies show that the abnormal person finds it more difficult to stand the stresses of legal abortion.[23] Such being the case, we may surmise that those women who are completely comfortable with abortions granted for psychological reasons may, in fact, have been in a better psychological condition than they thought.

In the fifth place, a woman's total social situation may point to the necessity for an abortion. The line, however, between true needs and brain-created ones is so fine that caution is in order. And the cautious person reflects upon a Japanese statistic: Of abortions performed, only 17 percent were for health reasons; all others pertained to worries about household finances.[24] Does a family's plan to buy a camper necessitate termination of an unplanned pregnancy? On the other hand, is the presence of a color television set in a slum home sufficient evidence that the family truly can afford this child? Perhaps television is the only bringer of cheer into drab surroundings. It is easy to pass judgment with dilated eyes and to miss subtleties. Will a new baby deprive a gifted brother of the opportunity for appropriate training? How will that brother feel about his education when he learns that its cost was the reason for aborting a younger sister or brother he longed for? There may be true needs which necessitate cutting the monkey-rope, but I suspect that they are fewer in number than proponents of abortion on demand claim.

Finally, there is the possibility of fetal deformity. Nearly half of the liveborn children of mothers who have German measles during the first four weeks of pregnancy will have defects, such as deafness, cataracts in the eyes, and heart abnormalities.[25] Techniques are being perfected which enable physicians to predict with considerable certainty that the child, if born, will be abnormal. If such a prediction is made, does it establish necessity for abortion?

There is much in the Old Testament view of life that supports an affirmative answer. We noted that "four are compared with a dead man: the lame, the blind, the leper and the childless."[26]

There would seem to be no demand to give life to beings who would be as good as dead. Flesh that has no possiblity for giving visibility to the breath of life does not require unqualified reverence. The New Testament, on the other hand, is just as interested in the persons who surround a deformed child as in that child himself. Does he draw forth from them a fullness of love that would not be elicited by a normal baby? Does he constitute for the parents, as many a cripple did for Jesus, the opportunity to make clear what God's love for "the stranger" is like?

From the point of view of Beethoven's parents, his conception was a tragedy. The histories of their previous children pointed to the strong possibility of his being abnormal. The father was not a stable family man. The mother was worn out. An abortion, if it had been available, would have brought relief. Yet how tragic for the world if that flesh had been denied the possibility of writing the "Hymn to Joy"!

Because the tragic dimension is so close to the surface, we must be cautious. In some instances, it would be tragic not to abort. Parents can be choked by the monkey-rope binding them to an abnormal offspring. At other times it would be tragic to abort. Parental love can be purest when there is no possibility that "the stranger" in their midst will satisfy any of their desires. To both of these possibilities must be added the tragedy of uncertainty. Tests only point to probabilities. The decision to cut or not to cut the monkey-rope must be made now. And it must be made without full knowledge of what the parents can endure and of what the child will bring. It is impossible to discern all the monkey-ropes that will tug at the lives involved through the years.

The foregoing analysis affirms that there are occasions when it is necessary to cut the monkey-rope binding child to mother. These times come much less frequently than advocates of abortion on demand assume, but more frequently than those who categorically oppose abortion believe. It is never, however, crystal clear when the decision for an abortion is the right decision.

What is clear is that abortion is not a woman's *right*. Abortion is not something a woman can demand as a woman. To speak of abortion as a *right* is to assume that flesh is not tied to spirit. It is to believe that the essential self is not committed to the fleshly consequences of fleshly acts. Since that position has been rejected as a distortion of the biblical view of man, it follows that there is no *right* to abortion within a monkey-rope concept of life.

Neither is abortion a *just* action or the *most loving* thing to do. To employ such language is to imply more insight than we have. It is also to skate perilously close to the thin ice of hypocrisy. We may deem it necessary to cut the monkey-rope, to cut life adrift, but we cannot be sure that an action so drastic is *just*. From a larger perspective, it might appear a most unjust decision. Melville speaks of

> Things hard to prove: decorum's wile,
> Malice discreet, judicious guile;
> Good done with ill intent...
> And hate under life's fair hue
> Prowls like the shark in sunned Pacific blue.[27]

Because we are dealing with flesh that has the potential for imaging the Creator's purpose, I hold back from using words suggesting that there can be taking of life which is not tragic.

Secondly, Christ said that there is no greater love than that involved in laying down one's life for another. At best, then, the taking of life is of a lesser order. It may be loving in the situation, but it is not the *most loving* thing to do. Abortion may seem to be the lesser of two evils. It can be a means for preserving other claims upon one's love, just as permitting a man to drown can be necessary in order to go on caring for one's family. But to say that either is the *most loving* decision is to leap over the fence which separates our knowledge from that of God.

9. EUTHANASIA

While involuntarily living among the cannibals of the Typee valley, Herman Melville happened one day upon a canoe in which sat the wooden likeness of a native warrior. He saw

> the warrior, holding his paddle with both hands in the act of rowing, leaning forward and inclining his head, as if eager to hurry on his voyage. Glaring at him for ever, and face to face, was a polished human skull, which crowned the prow of the canoe. The spectral figurehead, reversed in its position, glancing backwards, seemed to mock the impatient attitude of the warrior.[1]

Row as fast as you will, your death is always looking you in the eye.

If Melville had chanced to cross the Spreuer Bridge in Lucerne, he might have added that death walks up to us at the least expected moment. Above the heads of those who stroll across that bridge are painted scenes of the Dance of Death. A skeleton is best man as a couple marry. Another helps a merchant to load his ship. At an altar a priest is assisted by a skeleton in the robes of a deacon.

From the South Seas and Switzerland comes the message that death is to be reckoned with but not controlled. We cannot put off its approach or hasten its coming. That is the common understanding, but Queequeg thought differently. He decided he was dying and ordered the ship's carpenter to build his coffin. When it was ready, he lay in it to check the fit. Onlookers expected him to die then and there. Suddenly he rallied and, in substance, said, that the cause of his sudden convalescence was this;—at a critical moment, he had just recalled a little duty ashore, which he was leaving undone; and therefore had changed his mind about dying: he could not die yet, he averred. They asked him, then, whether to live or die was a matter of his own sovereign will and pleasure. He answered, certainly.[2]

In a Vienna clinic, experimental subjects were hypnotized. A state of happiness was suggested. When tested, there was an increased amount in their blood of an agent effective against typhoid fever. The same persons, when told to feel sad, had greatly reduced resistance to infection.[3]

Do such findings imply that the care of a physician is not to be sought? Because our spirits are capable of tugging at the monkey-rope and pulling the flesh out of the jaws of illness, is medical care unnecessary? Is medicine a brain-created need? No. Such a line of reasoning is neither scientific nor Christian. It severs flesh from the breath of life. Although mental attitudes do affect the flesh, it is also true that the condition of the flesh can lift up or pull down the spirit. Modern medicine confers blessings. No one would want to return to the age of Montaigne when physicians were unable to remove kidney stones. And the great essayist's stoic indifference to those stones did not cause them to dissolve. Flesh has maladies that mind is unable to master.

The care of a doctor is to be sought in times of illness and for regular checkups. If the care of a physician is to be sought, does that mean that everything that is medically possible is to be done? Are we obligated to acquiesce in the employment of every known *means* for dealing with the diagnosed problem? On the contrary, all things possible are not necessarily beneficial. Subtle-mindedness is in order. It is appropriate to differentiate between *ordinary* and *extraordinary* means for dealing with illness.

A medical technique is *ordinary* if it is reasonable in the light of the sufferer's total condition. *Yes* answers from the physician, the patient, and his family to three questions establish the wisdom of a procedure: (1) Will the recommended treatment, medication, or operation support a life that is worth living? (2) Is the cost of what is proposed bearable? (3) Will the health that is preserved enable the patient to fulfill obligations to his family, his community, and God?

Although these questions are seldom asked explicitly in the consulting room, they do undergird the reasonableness of most medical care. The majority of proposed treatments, drugs, and surgical procedures are *ordinary* means for preserving health. They help to maintain delight in living and devotion to one's neighbors and God. Where, then, do we draw the line between these means and *extraordinary* ones? It is difficult to draw. The late American man of letters Edmund Wilson refused to use a hearing aid, and he would not submit to having a pacemaker installed. Both devices are thought ordinary in most circles. Since Wilson, who had a remarkably subtle mind, thought them extraordinary, we must ponder his reasons.

Apparently Edmund Wilson felt that a pacemaker would keep his heart beating without guaranteeing him worthwhile life. He had lived to write. His work was accomplished. All that he had to say was in print. He had fulfilled his obligations as he conceived them. Why use an artificial mechanism in the chest to keep his heart beating regularly when his heart was not in the physical existence that would thereby be maintained?

Let us try now to define an *extraordinary* means for preserving life. (1) It is a treatment or drug or operation which offers little or no possibility of success in maintaining worthwhile living. Even if the heart is kept beating, the patient does not benefit significantly. (2) The price is not right if it is in direct conflict with the values for which a person has lived. Wilson lived to write; only secondarily did he write to live. Therefore, a pacemaker which would only support physical existence, whatever its cost, was too expensive. Or, consider a person who has given himself unstintingly to others. If medical care will be destructively costly to those he loves, it is extraordinary in nature. (3) Life is not an end in itself. It is given by God so that the recipient may live for God and his fellowmen. When that obligation has been carried out, when one has "set his house in order" (see 2 Kings 20:1), then techniques for extending life may be deemed extraordinary, especially when life has lost its savor and when the costs are prohibitive.

These guidelines can be applied to hemodialysis, the filtering of waste products out of the blood by means of the kidney machine. This treatment takes from six to fifteen hours and must be repeated several times a week. Costs range from $20,000 to $40,000 per year. From the point of view of medical technology, the kidney machine—once an extraordinary means—is ordinary, being used every day in major hospitals.

What about the patient's point of view? Hemodialysis is an ordinary means for the preservation of life if it does just that: if it sustains a productive life in which obligations are carried out, and if that life is preserved at a cost which is not catastrophic. It becomes extraordinary when the life of the sufferer comes to revolve around the machine to the exclusion of all else. Four years ago, Don Shevlin was on the verge of completing his Ph.D. degree. Then he went into kidney failure. Hemodialysis is keeping him alive, but he says: "I see myself as perennially pauperized." The degree not granted, no prospects for a teaching position, his savings wiped out, Shevlin lives on welfare payments of $178 a month, while the state of California pays $36,000 a year for his treatments.[4] Medical care is extraordinary when the maintenance of life is painful and costly, and when the living that is maintained is a slow dying.

If the distinction between ordinary and extraordinary means of preserving life can be made—and it *can* be made, although it must not be made with dilated eyes—why is it a fact that it is often ignored? Extraordinary means are employed when not demanded by the patient's total condition. Why is a living which is really a dying prolonged? Why is every means used when the circumstances suggest that some things ought *not* to be done? There are three parts to that question's answer.

First of all, we turn to physicians. They are taught to preserve life. They feel themselves bound by monkey-ropes to their patients. When death cuts that cord, the doctor feels defeated. He asks himself whether he could have done more. Was some stone left unturned, some means untried?

Coupled with this fear of professional failure is the physician's own fear of dying. Studies indicate that doctors are more afraid of death than control groups of their patients.[5] Psychiatrist Herman Feifel thinks this dread is a subconscious motive leading many into a profession which strives to conquer little deaths as well as the big one.[6]

London physician Alexander Comfort calls attention to the fact that the roots of the medical profession are in shamanism. The earliest doctor was the Shaman, one of whose claims to fame was his asserted ability to harrow hell. He could go to the realm of the dead, return unharmed, and sometimes retrieve one of its inhabitants.[7] Imitating their forerunners, modern doctors strive to harrow hell, to fight against death with no holds barred, to wrestle the dying from the jaws of Sheol.

As we noted in chapter 4, such rage against the realm of the dead is unnecessary. Christ harrowed hell, thus proclaiming that death does not cut the monkey-rope binding man to God. Because death is a God-defeated enemy, we need not fight it with mind and heart and might. What has been overcome by God can be welcomed as a friend. The Christian is therefore critical of those medical practitioners who insist upon using every means available for prolonging physical existence. From confidence in the resurrection of Jesus Christ flows criticism of that doctor who insists on doing everything possible to prolong life.

Roland Stevens, M.D., said in an address delivered on February 4, 1971:

> The effectiveness of medical technology has outstripped the quality of the professional conscience which guides it. Sometimes the professional conscience must be critically examined and the doctor be taught that what he can and what he should do, in this matter of deferring death, are not always the same.[8]

In the second place, the patient's family may insist that every means, ordinary and extraordinary, be pressed into service to prolong dying. The motive can be mercenary. Some states levy a tax on gifts made within three years of death. Beneficiaries of such gifts may ask the physician to do all in his power to keep the patient breathing so as to evade the tax collector. More often guilt is the motivating factor. Faced with the death of a loved one, one may experience an outbreak of hitherto imprisoned memories. What child has not, in a moment of anger, wished for a parent's death? There is also the old gag so true to life. A reporter interviewing a couple on their golden wedding anniversary asked: "Did you ever consider divorce?" And the reply: "Divorce, no; murder, yes!" In addition to these guilty thoughts, there is the guilt associated with recollections of deeds left undone. Remembrance of sins of omission and commission prompts family members to urge the doctor to use his skill for maintaining life. Where once they erred by doing too little, now they err by demanding too much of the physician. In the past they turned living into hell for their "loved one." Now, when that person's living is yielding to dying, they make the hell more harrowing by ordering treatments that are impelled by guilt masquerading as love.

Third, the patient often asks the physician to keep on trying. Because of the doctor-patient monkey-rope, that request is granted. It is understandable that a medical consultant would be reluctant to deny a sufferer's request, even when he knows that nothing successful can be done.

In her study of the stages through which a dying person passes (denial, anger, bargaining, depression, and resignation), Doctor Elisabeth Kübler-Ross found that *hope* is the one attitude that persists.[9] This hope may attach itself to the discovery of a wonder drug or to the possibility of being chosen for a promising experiment. It waits for the physician to appear at the sickroom door, medical journal in hand, with an announcement of the discovery of an effective treatment. The patient clings to each extraordinary means for prolonging living (or dying) that is offered.

Such grasping for straws is not necessary for the Christian. He believes that his dying has been caught up in the death and resurrection of Jesus Christ. As birth is a gift of God, so is death. Therefore, the Christian is not bound to strive officiously to prolong that living which is truly dying. Christ harrowed hell. Death does not cut the man-God monkey-rope. Hence, it is not obligatory to fetch hell into the hospital room by prolonging the agony of dying. The doctor may permit death to enter as a conquered enemy who is now to be greeted as a friend.

Disrespect for the flesh often accompanies the no-holds-barred warfare against dying which we have just criticized. While a brain-created need to prolong life is being pursued, true needs of the flesh are ignored. Flesh is not given its due. In the light of the four functions of the flesh described in chapter 2, how is proper respect to be shown to dying flesh?[10]

The first function of the flesh is to enable the breath of life to exercise control. Strength is a steady gait, a firm handclasp. Mastery means controlling one's voice in such fashion as to control others. Illness brings the loss of some of these fleshly powers.

The sick person feels weak. He is unable to help himself. In his helplessness, the dying person senses a foretaste of death's utter weakness.

Many medical procedures accentuate the fact that one's hand has lost its grip. The person, too, is losing his grip on life. Physicians speak of "managing" a patient. They take his care into their capable hands, thus confirming how incapable he is of managing his own affairs. He is connected to machines that live for him and to monitors that enable others to think for him. In short, flesh is denied the opportunity to continue expressing spirit. What it will lose in death is taken away in advance by those who assert that they are warding off dying.

What can be done to counter this trend? The patient can be given as much control as possible over his medical care. Perhaps he has previously expressed his thinking in the words of The Euthanasia Educational Fund's *Living Will:*

> If there is no reasonable expectation of my recovery from physical or mental disability, I, _____, request that I be allowed to die and not be kept alive by artificial means or heroic measures. Death is as much a reality as birth, growth, maturity and old age—it is the one certainty. I do not fear death as much as I fear the indignity of deterioration, dependence and hopeless pain. I ask that drugs be mercifully administered to me for terminal suffering even if they hasten the moment of death.[11]

Such a request should be honored. It gives the patient assurance that he is still "managing" his life.

Second, flesh is what brings the outside world inside. Eyes see, ears hear, noses smell; and, because they do, the spirit is aware of colors, sounds, and odors. These disclosures of the external world are clouded by illness, a problem which is aggravated by some medical practices. The patient often finds himself in colorless surroundings. Hospitals are ringed by parking lots, not flower gardens. Operating rooms are sterile, free from living microorganisms, but also barren. Intensive care units are mechanically efficient but humanly deficient.

The poet Yeats once said: "I like a little seaweed in my definition of water."[12] H_2O seemed to Yeats an abstract, lifeless definition. He wanted seaweed entangled in his toes when he went swimming. Following upon that thought, how can we make certain that the *seaweed* is not removed from the environment of the dying person? We can, first of all, keep him at home as long as possible. Medical efficiency does not always compensate for the loss of familiar sights. Then, when an institutional setting becomes necessary, there ought to be provision for items to which memory clings: favorite foods, plants, pictures, but especially the loved faces themselves. All too soon the senses lose their powers. But, before they do, we must not eliminate the odors, sounds, and colors on which they feed. It is no blessing to prolong dying in such fashion that the patient is forcefully reminded of what death is like.

In the third place, flesh is where one's breath of life is made visible for others. I express myself in and through the fleshly contractions of my face. Gestures reveal spirit. So do those spurts of air we call "speech." Illness may render flesh inexpressive. A stroke tightens the side of a face, blurs speech, and paralyzes a hand. Medical procedures may make such weaknesses of the flesh more frightening. Drugs and machines, while offering some benefits, further limit the flesh's potential for bodying-forth the breath of life.

What is to be done? Flesh is to be treated with respect. It must be kept clean. As control of bodily functions ebbs, linens are to be changed regularly and gentle baths given. Whenever possible, rituals of eating should be preserved. Important to eating are taste and color and companionship. Intravenous infusions of nutrients are effective and efficient, but they are like water without seaweed. A spoonful of food in a human hand, if any way feasible, is so much better. Flesh that has expressed personality is to be yielded the honor due the spirit. Till death they are linked by a monkey-rope.

Even after death, flesh is to receive loving care. It is disrespectful to make up a dead body to look like a living one. Living flesh expresses the spirit; dead flesh expresses nothing. It is what remains when the spirit has departed. To forget that distinction, or to use cosmetics to cover it over, is to do flesh no honor. More of spirit is revealed in flesh pinched by agony than in a corpse "restored" to some similitude of peaceful slumber. Therefore, a dead body should be cleansed lovingly, wrapped in cloth, and returned to the dust.

Finally, flesh makes relationship possible. As illness advances, so does separation from loved ones. Dying is a solitary affair at best. Doctors heighten the horror by increasing isolation. The expiring patient may be attached to all types of cords except the one he most needs: the monkey-rope binding him to other human beings. Therefore, the preservation of community is essential. Where the alternatives are tender loving care or medical efficiency, there is no choice. Better to die in the arms of a loved one than in the embrace of a machine.

Community is also destroyed by mendacity. Man is tied to man by the monkey-rope of truth. As we have seen, there are times when it is necessary to cut that rope. However, unless such times are kept to a minimum, integrity disappears from human relationships. That is the situation in which the medical profession finds itself today.

Too often doctors have been situationalists. Too often have they withheld the truth from patients. They have told lies so frequently to the terminally ill that relationship has been shattered. They have been caught in these deceptions, and they are no longer trusted. Time and again as a pastor I have visited patients who expressed doubts concerning the report given them by the surgeon. "He told me they found no cancer, but that's what they told ——, when actually they sewed him up because the cancer was too far gone." Such mendacity cuts the monkey-rope of truth just when the dying person most needs to have confidence in his physician.

Experience shows that most terminally ill persons *sense* their condition. So it would be preferable for the doctor to speak honestly. He can give simple information in response to the patient's questions. At the same time, he can hold out to the person with whom he is linked some grounds for hope.

It is vital for the dying person's family and his physician to draw close to him in his dying. Soon enough relationship will be broken. Therefore, to break it prematurely is an act of abandonment. It is to cut the monkey-rope of truth and love. The one cut adrift slides into the jaws of despair.

Our argument so far suggests that it is better to care for the flesh and to allow the person to die in some dignity than to strive *officiously* to keep a dying person alive when the means employed to that end offer no real possibility of success. It is wrong to treat a healthy person as if he were terminally ill. It is equally wrong to treat a dying person as if he had years of meaningful life ahead of him. Paul Ramsey reminds us that:

> To say "there is no other hope" does not mean that there is no other *choice*. Men as men need not choose survival under any or all conditions. Faced with some sorts of elective life, death may become more electable still and more consonant with human dignity.[13]

To let a person have a good death is to decline to employ means that would be *extraordinary* in his case. For a person suffering from terminal cancer, even intravenous feeding can be extraordinary. It might be better to give what nourishment is acceptable by mouth, reduce pain as much as possible, and permit the sufferer to expire. Of course, such a decision must be made by the doctor and the patient's family in harmony with the sufferer's will if expressed.

Such assertions require us to define death more carefully As we saw in chapter 3, breathing and heartbeat are the traditional signs of life. When they are absent, death is present. An electroencephalogram (EEG) is now used to indicate brain life or death. A flat reading shows the cessation of electrical activitity in the brain. Is such a reading by itself sufficient to define death? No. After the brain is dead, as defined by an EEG, the heart can go on beating naturally for some time. Breathing is more closely tied to electrical activity in the brain. Spontaneous respiratory activity stops soon after brain death. Then, when the heart is no longer being nourished by oxygen, it too fails. Of course, both heart and lung activity can be sustained by a respirator.

Because the line between life and death is not crystal clear, reverence for life demands a maximal rather than a minimal definition of death. In this case, the minimum is the electroencephalogram. The maximum is brain death plus the inability of heart and lungs to function spontaneously. If respiratory and circulatory activity are being maintained only by medical technology and the brain is dead, then it is appropriate to turn off the respirator and declare the patient dead.

Thus far we have been speaking about letting a person die when nothing that can be done offers hope for preserving a life worth living. What now about the person whose "worthless" life is preserved by food, water, and simple drugs in contrast with extraordinary means? Consider the man who named the animals and plants, not Adam, but Linnaeus. His classifying organ, his brain, was damaged by a stroke. First, he forgot his great book, *The System of Nature*. Then he could not remember what he was called. The man who named his fellow creatures forgot his own name.[14]

It is hard to imagine that life for Linnaeus was worth living. He lived to classify. When he was no longer able to classify even himself, would it not have been in order to grant him a peaceful death? Since euthanasia means a "good death," would it not have been good to give him a poisonous drink?

But I am unwilling to cross that which is for me a narrow but deep divide. It is one thing to refuse to prolong dying. Heroic measures are unnecessary. When there is no hope other than in extraordinary means, there is another choice. Not everything must be done that can be done. If the brain is dead and the respirator is the only thing that will keep heart and lungs going, use of the machine is not obligatory. If the person would die of cancer almost immediately if intravenous feeding were withdrawn, the next bottle is not required. In these cases, the patient is permitted to die. It is quite another thing to take some positive action which produces death: poison or injecting a bubble of air into the bloodstream. To kill when nothing more unusual than food, water, and simple drugs are sustaining life is to assume that we know with assurance the point where hope disappears.

In a letter to *The National Observer*, Paul P. Krikorian, M.D., writes:

> When I am sure there is *absolutely no hope*, then I refuse to sustain life by artificial, mechanical means. But let me add that to be sure there is no hope can be quite difficult in some cases. I have a patient who is enjoying life, with his wife and children now, with very little residual disability, who was a total vegetable for over 30 days, in a coma from a cerebral thrombosis 11 years ago![15]

Because the chasm between life and death is narrow but deep, it is best neither to prolong artificially the life of the dying nor to induce artificially the death of the living. When life is sustained by food, water, and medications, such life is to be maintained. It is wrong for a healthy person to starve himself to death. It can also be wrong to force intravenous feeding upon a dying person. But is it right to give poison to a person who appears to be dying, yet whose life is sustained by nutrients taken by mouth and who requires no linkages to machines? I do not think it right, for two reasons.

Some of the consequences of suicide may follow upon that type of euthanasia which involves direct taking of life. We recall the suicide of John Berryman described in chapter 4. In that act of despair, Berryman was tied by a monkey-rope to his father, who had shot himself when John was twelve. That father thought that his life was without worth, yet it had value to his son. That child's candle of faith was blown out when his father snuffed out his. John Berryman felt bound by a monkey-rope to his father's suicide. When the sire slipped, the son slid.

Berryman's is not an isolated case. Timothy Foote writes:

> The more people hear suicide discussed as an honorable solution to the pangs of living, the more people—given other stresses—are likely to try it. It is statistically true that if anyone in a child's close-knit world commits suicide, the child's chances of eventually doing the same thing increase by as much as 75%.[16]

If more and more people talk about positive euthanasia (concrete action to take life) as "an honorable solution" to the problem of a declining life that is maintained by ordinary means, then more and more people are likely to try it. That being the case, we can expect the lives of others who are bound to them to be affected. From the point of view of the individual, life may be so pointless as to indicate termination. Yet that person is tied by monkey-ropes to others who draw the point of their living from his life. If they interpret his act as a lack of faith, as John Berryman did his father's suicide, then their candles of faith may be blown out.

Second, I cannot sanction positive euthanasia because life is not absolutely at one's own disposal. Life is God's gift. There remains, therefore, a place for man to stand aside and permit God to do the taking of life. It is wrong to strive to hold onto a life that God is taking. It is also wrong to take a life that God is not calling. Such language does not take back all that was said in the beginning of this chapter about seeking medical care. It is not a return to that attitude which says that God operates through *natural* causes and that, therefore, to interfere with nature's course is to go against the stream of God's will. On the contrary, the intelligence that makes medicine possible is a good gift of God. It is to be used within the limits already noted to preserve life and health. But there are fences. We do not know with God-like precision the boundary between life and death. We do not know when Omniscience knows that there is no hope. Hence, we grant to *nature* the role of preserving us from presumption. If nature is certainly taking life and our best efforts will do no more than prolong dying, then we may appropriately halt the extraordinary means. If, on the other hand, nature is preserving life, even though the life that is lived is as tragic as Linnaeus', then we must hold back from officiously taking it.

If there is nothing that we can *do* in such instances to hasten dying, is there a way we can *behave* if we are the persons dying? Giving-in-dying remains a possibility for Christ's followers. Instead of a lingering death posing a problem, it can be transformed into a gift of love. A man's mortal illness is the last thing uniquely his own that a dying man has to give. Perhaps his disease can be of help to researchers. What is learned from evaluating it may constitute a gift of love to others. Before we reach such a pass, we can indicate that we are willing to give our dying in such fashion for the benefit of others.

This possibility does not justify all research on the dying, however. If the experiments are not related to the specific malady of the dying person, then he ought not be asked to participate—or others ought not give their consent if he cannot—in a project where the one last thing he has to offer, his dying, makes no difference. The research project must be specifically tied to the illness, or it lacks fleshy concreteness for the patient.

We also can behave toward our dying as Fred Harris did. Early in 1972, doctors informed Harris that he had inoperable cancer of both lungs. A number of periodicals reported on what this Beverly Hills, California, realtor did next. He visited gun shops. He went to the city morgue to look at the bodies of suicides. And he brooded. Then a friend asked Harris to call upon an acquaintance hospitalized with lung cancer. After that visit, Harris realized that both he and the patient felt better. He had given what was his—his feelings about his own hopeless malignancy—to one who most needed that gift. As a dying man, he spoke to a dying man about death. The result was lessened apprehension.

What if both of these ways of behaving are denied us? There is, finally, the potential of dying flesh for revealing God. It can be the place where God becomes visible. This possibility was not understood by Albrecht Dürer when he was young and healthy. He painted a portrait of himself in 1500. By the way he fashioned it, he made clear that he was using Christ to advertise Dürer. The artist posed himself in a posture frequently associated with Christ. His right hand mimics the gesture of blessing of the *Savior of the World*. He has even altered his features to make them conform to those of Christ in traditional portrayals. He depicted himself as Christ to emphasize the impact that he intended Albrecht Dürer to have on the world. Dürer felt that strong, healthy flesh was the place where the creativity of God is made visible.

Looking at this portrait, we realize that it does not reveal the love of God in Christ. It is a picture of human pride, not of the power of God made perfect in human weakness. That nobler theme was realized by the dying Dürer in a self-portrait of 1522. In it he reversed the former situation. Christ is drawn in the likeness of a suffering Dürer. His body is ravaged by a lingering illness. Dürer is a broken man. Yet he makes of his pain and physical decay a gift: the gift of a reminder that God's love became visible in the beaten and broken body of Christ. When Jesus was being edged out of the world on a cross, when he was dying, then—as never before when he was hale and hearty—was the love of God revealed. When there was nothing more to do, Jesus behaved in such a way that his suffering was transparent to the love of God.

CONCLUDING NOTE: MONKEY-ROPES

Sport was her name, and her home was our front-yard tree. Among its branches her children played. In one of its rotten holes, she nursed her squirrel babies. One day, those officials who worry about decaying trees sent out the demolition crew. Sport's home was reduced to a pile of fireplace logs. She despaired on the stump. She jumped, trying to clamber up tractionless air, remembering that her babies were somewhere up there. And she became a link between Loren Eiseley and me.

In writing this book, I have felt a monkey-rope binding me to Professor Eiseley. My report to him on Sport established a personal bond, but it was nearly a decade ago that his writings began to open my eyes to the glories and tragedies of our monkey-rope world. My words are shamed by the lyric quality of his; yet they limp along knowing that words can dance when the caller is Loren Eiseley. To him, therefore, I stand indebted. Credit is given in the footnotes, but here I wish to thank him for calling my attention to *Kamongo* and for thoughts too numerous to cite that shaped my thinking.

Professor Paul Ramsey responded to my first paper on abortion with helpful criticism. His books are models of step-by-step ethical analysis. Where my reasoning is logical, I am grateful to him. But I must cut the monkey-rope that would implicate him in my slips. His critique of my manuscript was searching, but he is not to be held accountable for this book.

I am in debt to Doctors Jean and Frank Johnston. They

checked with care the medical data used by me and saved me, more than once, from the sharp teeth of error. Because I am tied to them by the doctor-patient monkey-rope, I have come to judge other physicians by their high standards of wisdom and goodness.

Although their names are not mentioned in the text, Charles S. Bartolett, Dale E. Owens, J. Dennis Williams, Robert H. Wright, and Charles Yrigoyen, Jr., are linked to me by monkey-ropes woven through years of meeting monthly to discuss books. They have read this work in typescript and made me aware of loose connections.

Lacking the devoted skill of Mrs. George D. Braun, I could not have slipped the work of writing into my pastoral schedule. She is the kind of secretary who delights the perfectionist. Mrs. Braun has been ready to type the same pages time and again, thus enabling me to go on worrying about the content and style of this book.

Our children, Anne Gray and Peter John, have been linked to a father who was home writing but not at home for them. May they forgive! The role of my wife is suggested by the words of the dedication.

The monkey-ropes binding me to these Ishmaels, and many others, pulled me from the jaws of the shark of error that "glides white through the phosphorus sea."[1] The image is Melville's, and I give thanks for his life and works to the God who presides over the miraculous emergence of such men.

JOHN GALEN MCELLHENNEY

Wynnewood, Pennsylvania
Thanksgiving Day, 1972

NOTES

NOTES FOR CHAPTER ONE

1 Herman Melville, *Moby Dick* (New York: Holt, Rinehart & Winston, Inc., 1948), pp. 317-318.
2 Henry David Thoreau, *Walden* (New York: The Heritage Press, 1939), p. 32.
3 Laurence M. Gould, "Antarctica: The World's Greatest Laboratory," *The American Scholar*, vol. 40, no. 3 (Summer, 1971), pp. 408-409.
4 Jeanne Wellenkamp, "The Cardinal Meets Vivaldi," *The Christian Science Monitor*, July 9, 1971.

NOTES FOR CHAPTER TWO

1 Herman Melville, *Moby Dick* (New York: Holt, Rinehart & Winston, Inc., 1948), p. 466.
2 *Ibid.*, pp. 126-127.
3 See Roland de Vaux, *Ancient Israel* (London: Darton, Longman & Todd, 1961), pp. 21-22.
4 *Interpreter's Dictionary of the Bible* (Nashville: Abingdon Press, 1962), vol. 1, p. 715.
5 de Vaux, *op. cit.*, p. 41.
6 *Ibid.*, p. 56.
7 *The Christian Science Monitor*, December 3, 1971.
8 *Ibid.*, January 14, 1972.

NOTES FOR CHAPTER THREE

1 Craig Karpel, "Immortality Is Fully Deductible," *Playboy*, October, 1971, p. 150.
2 See Joachim Jeremias, *New Testament Theology* (London: SCM Press, Ltd., 1971), vol. 1, p. 284.
3 See Bernard Häring, *The Law of Christ* (Westminster, Maryland: The Newman Press, 1966), vol. 3, p. 205.

4 For the outline that follows, I have consulted the following works: John F. Dedek, *Human Life: Some Moral Issues* (New York: Sheed & Ward, Inc., 1972), pp. 60-63; Andre E. Hellegers, "Fetal Development," *Theological Studies*, vol. 31, no. 1 (March, 1970), pp. 3-9; Paul Ramsey, "Reference Points in Deciding About Abortion," *The Morality of Abortion*, ed. John T. Noonan, Jr. (Cambridge: Harvard University Press, 1970), pp. 64-79; and "Life Before Birth," Life Educational Reprint 27, reprinted from *Life*, April 30, 1965.

5 Paul Ramsey, "Reference Points in Deciding about Abortion," *The Morality of Abortion*, pp. 75f. (Italics in original)

6 See *The Interpreter's Dictionary of the Bible* (Nashville: Abingdon Press, 1962), vol. 3, p. 10.

7 Michel de Montaigne, *Essays*, trans. J. M. Cohen (New York: Penguin Books, Inc., 1958), p. 375.

8 *Ibid.*, pp. 376f.

9 W. Dorland, *American Pocket Medical Dictionary* (Philadelphia: W. B. Saunders Company, 1953), p. 307.

10 *The Merck Manual of Diagnosis and Therapy* (Merck Sharp & Dohme Research Laboratories, 1966), p. 626.

11 *Ibid.*, p. 627.

12 Montaigne, *op. cit.*, p. 376.

13 *Ibid.*, pp. 380f.

14 Lawrence Mosher, "When There Is No Hope . . . Why Prolong Life?", *The National Observer*, March 4, 1972.

15 For the following outline of Hebrew funeral customs, I am indebted to Roland de Vaux, *Ancient Israel* (London: Darton, Longman & Todd, 1961), pp. 56-61; for the framework of interpretation, I am indebted to Arnold van Gennep, *The Rites of Passage* (Chicago: The University of Chicago Press, 1960), pp. 146-165.

16 de Vaux, *op. cit.*, p. 60.

NOTES FOR CHAPTER FOUR

1 Constantine FitzGibbon, *The Life of Dylan Thomas* (Boston: Little, Brown and Company, 1965), p. 164.

2 *The Poems of Dylan Thomas*, edited with an Introduction and Notes by Daniel Jones (New York: A New Directions Book, 1971), pp. 207f.

3 Joachim Jeremias, *New Testament Theology* (London: SCM Press, Ltd., 1971), p. 104.

4 Herman Melville, *Moby Dick* (New York: Holt, Rinehart & Winston, Inc., 1948), p. 333.

5 Michel de Montaigne, *Essays* (New York: Penguin Books, Inc., 1958), p. 377.

6 *Ibid.*, p. 389.

7 Émile Mâle, *Religious Art from the Twelfth to the Eighteenth Century* (New York: Pantheon Books, Inc., 1949), p. 55.

8 Jeremias, *op. cit.*, p. 306.

9 *The Interpreter's Dictionary of the Bible* (Nashville: Abingdon Press, 1962), vol. 1, p. 854.

10 See Jeremias, *op. cit.*, pp. 75 and 129.

11 See Michael Gough, *The Early Christians* (New York: Frederick A. Praeger, 1961), pp. 83f.

NOTES FOR CHAPTER FIVE

1 Homer W. Smith, *Kamongo or, The Lungfish and the Padre* (New York: The Viking Press, 1956). Copyright 1932, 1949, © 1960 by Homer W. Smith. Reprinted by permission of The Viking Press, Inc.
2 *Ibid.*, pp. 67f.
3 *Ibid.*, p. 85.
4 *The Christian Science Monitor*, December 7, 1971.
5 Paul Ramsey, *The Patient As Person* (New Haven: Yale University Press, 1970), pp. 245-246.
6 *Ibid.*, p. 248.
7 Loren Eiseley, *Francis Bacon and the Modern Dilemma* (Freeport, New York: Books for Libraries Press, 1970), pp. 63-65.
8 Henry Thoreau, *Walden* (New York: The Heritage Press, 1939), p. 324.
9 *Newsweek*, July 24, 1972, p. 74.
10 *The Christian Science Monitor*, May 23, 1972.
11 W. H. Auden, "Contra Blake," *Epistle to a Godson* (New York: Random House, Inc., 1972), p. 65.
12 *Christianity Today*, February 18, 1972, p. 44.
13 Richard Hofstadter, *America at 1750* (New York: Alfred A. Knopf, 1971), p. xi.
14 *Saturday Review*, March 11, 1972, p. 40.
15 *The Christian Science Monitor*, May 11, 1972.
16 Melville, *Moby Dick* (New York: Holt, Rinehart & Winston, Inc., 1948), p. 202.
17 *Ibid.*, p. 467.
18 Roger Shinn, "Survival Ethics Toward a Zero-Growth Economy," *Christianity and Crisis*, March 20, 1972, p. 56.
19 Dale White, ed., *Dialogue in Medicine and Theology* (Nashville: Abingdon Press, 1967), p. 46.
20 Melville, *op. cit.*, p. 329.
21 Smith, *op. cit.*, pp. 92f.

NOTES FOR CHAPTER SIX

1 Quoted in *Time*, January 10, 1972, p. 34.
2 Roland H. Bainton, *Erasmus of Christendom* (New York: Charles Scribner's Sons, 1969), p. 122.
3 Herman Melville, *Moby Dick* (New York: Holt, Rinehart & Winston, Inc., 1948), pp. 21 and 28.
4 *Ibid.*, p. 54.
5 *Ibid.*, p. 24.
6 *Ibid.*, p. 50.
7 *Ibid.*, p. 59.
8 "Playboy Interview: Saul Alinsky," *Playboy*, March, 1972, p. 62.
9 For the material that follows, I am indebted to Jacques Ellul, *Violence:*

Reflections from a Christian Perspective, trans. Celia Gaul Kings (New York: The Seabury Press, Inc., 1969), pp. 5ff.

[10] *The Christian Science Monitor,* December 31, 1971.

[11] Richard Hofstadter, *America at 1750* (New York: Alfred A. Knopf, 1971), p. 26.

[12] Joachim Jeremias, *New Testament Theology* (London: SCM Press, Ltd., 1971), p. 221.

[13] *Ibid.,* p. 222.

[14] *Saturday Review,* July 17, 1971, pp. 16-17.

[15] See Robert Bolt, *A Man for All Seasons* (New York: Random House, Inc., 1962), pp. 65-66.

NOTES FOR CHAPTER SEVEN

[1] Jacques Ellul, *Violence: Reflections from a Christian Perspective* (New York: The Seabury Press, Inc., 1969), pp. 94-97.

[2] *Ibid.,* p. 99.

[3] *The Christian Science Monitor,* December 15, 1971.

[4] Paul Verghese, "The I That Chooses," *The Christian Century,* June 7, 1972, p. 666.

[5] Richard Hofstadter, *America at 1750* (New York: Alfred A. Knopf, 1971), p. 123.

[6] *Selected Poems of Herman Melville,* ed. with an Introduction by Robert Penn Warren (New York: Random House, Inc., 1970), p. 93. (Italics in the original)

[7] *Ibid.,* p. 95.

[8] *Time,* May 1, 1972, p. 18.

[9] Verghese, *op. cit.,* p. 664.

[10] David Little, "On the 'Ethics of Principle,'" *The Christian Century,* December 8, 1971, p. 1442.

[11] Roland Bainton, *Erasmus of Christendom* (New York: Charles Scribner's Sons, 1969), p. 120.

[12] Rosemary Ruether and Fred Branfman, "A Liturgy from the Lands of Burning Children," *Christianity and Crisis,* June 26, 1972, p. 156.

[13] *Ibid.*

[14] Craig Karpel, "Immortality Is Fully Deductible," *Playboy,* October, 1971, p. 252.

[15] *Sacramentum Mundi: An Encyclopedia of Theology,* (New York: Herder and Herder, Inc., 1969), vol. 3, p. 314.

[16] Herman Melville, *Moby Dick* (New York: Holt, Rinehart & Winston, Inc., 1948), p. 226.

NOTES FOR CHAPTER EIGHT

[1] *Playboy,* February, 1972.

[2] R. F. R. Gardner, *Abortion: The Personal Dilemma* (Grand Rapids, Michigan; William B. Eerdmans Publishing Company, 1972), p. 13.

[3] George Santayana, *Reason in Society,* p. 35, quoted by Morton White, *Science and Sentiment in America* (New York: Oxford University Press, 1972), p. 258.

4 *The National Observer,* January 8, 1972.
5 *Time,* December 20, 1971, p. 51.
6 *The National Observer,* June 17, 1972.
7 John T. Noonan, Jr., ed., *The Morality of Abortion: Legal and Historical Perspectives* (Cambridge: Harvard University Press, 1970), p. 57.
8 Arnold van Gennep, *The Rites of Passage* (Chicago: The University of Chicago Press, 1960), p. 53.
9 Noonan, *op. cit.,* p. 76.
10 Loren Eiseley, *The Firmament of Time* (New York: Atheneum Publishers, 1962), pp. 28-29.
11 *Christianity Today,* March 17, 1972.
12 Dale White, ed., *Dialogue in Medicine and Theology* (Nashville: Abingdon Press, 1968), pp. 105f.
13 Gardner, *op. cit.,* p. 225.
14 Dale White, *op. cit.,* p. 102.
15 Gardner, *op. cit.,* p. 195.
16 *Ibid.,* p. 168.
17 *Ibid.,* p. 169.
18 *Ibid.*
19 Quoted in *ibid.,* p. 152.
20 *Ibid.,* p. 212. (Italics added by author)
21 *Ibid.,* p. 219.
22 *Ibid.,* p. 38.
23 *Ibid.,* p. 234.
24 *Ibid.,* p. 47.
25 *Ibid.,* p. 198.
26 Joachim Jeremias, *New Testament Theology* (London: SCM Press, Ltd., 1971), vol. 1, p. 104.
27 From "Clarel," *Selected Poems of Herman Melville* (New York: Random House, Inc., 1970), p. 238.

NOTES FOR CHAPTER NINE

1 Herman Melville, *Typee* (New York: Limited Editions Club, 1935), p. 273.
2 Herman Melville, *Moby Dick* (New York: Holt, Rinehart & Winston, Inc., 1948), p. 475.
3 Viktor E. Frankl, *The Doctor and the Soul,* rev. ed. (New York: Alfred A. Knopf, 1965), pp. 81f.
4 *Time,* December 20, 1971, p. 57.
5 Paul Ramsey, *The Patient as Person* (New Haven: Yale University Press, 1970), footnote on p. 3.
6 *The Philadelphia Inquirer Magazine,* March 19, 1972.
7 *Center for Democratic Institutions Report,* February, 1972.
8 Pamphlet distributed by The Euthanasia Educational Fund.
9 Elisabeth Kübler-Ross, *On Death and Dying* (New York: The Macmillan Company, 1970), p. 138.
10 In what follows I am indebted to Dr. William F. May for insights gained from reading his paper, "The Sacral Power of Death in Contemporary Experience," *Social Research,* vol. 39, no. 3 (Autumn, 1972), pp. 462-488.

[11] For further information, write to: The Euthanasia Educational Fund, 250 West 57th St., New York, NY 10019.

[12] Quoted by William F. May, "The Sacral Power of Death in Contemporary Experience," *Social Research*, vol. 39, no. 3 (Autumn, 1972), p. 481.

[13] Ramsey, *op. cit.*, p. 236 (Italics in the original).

[14] Loren Eiseley, *Darwin's Century* (Garden City, New York: Doubleday Anchor Books, 1958), pp. 25-26.

[15] *The National Observer*, April 1, 1972 (Italics in the original).

[16] *Time*, June 12, 1972, p. 85.

NOTE FOR CONCLUDING NOTE

[1] "Commemorative of a Naval Victory," *Selected Poems of Herman Melville* (New York: Random House, Inc., 1970), p. 152.

BJ
1533
.H9
M3
1973